ANXIETY AND DYSAUTONOMIA

ANXIETY AND DYSAUTONOMIA

Do I Have POTS or Autonomic Dysfunction?

The Mind-Body Wellness Program

(adapted from *Clinical Autonomic and Mitochondrial Disorders—Diagnosis, Prevention, and Treatment for Mind-Body Wellness*)

by
Nicholas L. DePace, MD, FACC,
Donald J. Parker, LCSW, and
Joseph Colombo, PhD, DNM, DHS

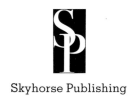

Skyhorse Publishing

Skyhorse Publishing books may be purchased in bulk at special discounts for sales promotion, corporate gifts, fund-raising, or educational purposes. Special editions can also be created to specifications. For details, contact the Special Sales Department, Skyhorse Publishing, 307 West 36th Street, 11th Floor, New York, NY 10018 or info@skyhorsepublishing.com.

Skyhorse® and Skyhorse Publishing® are registered trademarks of Skyhorse Publishing, Inc.®, a Delaware corporation.

Visit our website at www.skyhorsepublishing.com.

10 9 8 7 6 5 4 3 2 1

Library of Congress Cataloging-in-Publication Data is available on file.

Print ISBN: 978-1-5107-6090-5
eBook ISBN: 978-1-5107-6118-6

Cover design by Kai Texel

Printed in China

CONTENTS

(A D at the beginning of a table of content entry indicates a section specifically on the physician side (D for doctor); a P indicates a section specifically on the patient side)

CONTENT FORMAT

After the Introduction (including the Background, Mind-Body Wellness Program Basics, Parasympathetic and Sympathetic [P&S] monitoring, and Disclaimers), the main body of the book is written in two parts (see the next two pages as the example): one part to the patient or the patient's loved ones and one part to the physicians. The patient part is written on the right-hand page (the odd-numbered pages) and the physician part is written on the left-hand page (the even-numbered pages). Essentially the same information is presented in both parts, just using different styles ("languages") to communicate the information. In this way, patients (if interested) may see what the doctors may be, or as we believe should be, considering, and the physicians will have an example of a way of communicating with their patients, especially in this field that is poorly understood and even less well taught.

FOR PHYSICIANS

Most left-hand (or even-numbered) pages are written for physicians.

While other Dysautonomia books explain how to manage patients with autonomic dysfunction, we look to provide more information to help physicians treat autonomic dysfunction (aka, Dysautonomia). Furthermore, assuming no end organ damage or genetic causes, we believe the recommendations herein will help physicians to work with their patients to restore health and even wellness, if certain lifestyles are adopted.

This book will lean heavily toward supplements and lifestyle treatments for Anxiety and Dysautonomia. The primary reason is that there are only two pharmaceuticals (Midodrine and Northera) approved for autonomic dysfunction. All other pharmaceuticals that are recommended are off-label recommendations. In fact, there are now more supplements and lifestyles recommended in large, multi-center studies for Dysautonomia (including dosing; e.g., alpha-lipoic acid, fish oil, coenzyme Q10, and exercise) than approved pharmaceuticals.

Another reason is that, in our experience, by the time a patient sees us, they have been prescribed many mediations and in high dosages. Therefore, they have become intolerant or unresponsive to the few medications that we have found to work, but in very low dosages. The supplements and lifestyle modifications aid in enabling dosing of the pharmaceuticals in low or homeopathic dosages, and the pharmaceuticals are then able to help accelerate the relief brought about by the supplements and lifestyle modifications. In many cases, the goal is to eventually wean from the pharmaceuticals and maintain with lower-dose supplements and continued lifestyle modifications.

Continued on page 4 . . .

FOR PATIENTS AND THEIR LOVED ONES

Most right-hand (or odd-numbered) pages are written for patients.

While other Dysautonomia books explain how patients should live with autonomic dysfunction (aka, Dysautonomia), we look to help you to overcome your Dysautonomia and associated Anxiety. As we have helped countless numbers of patients in the past, we hope to help you to reclaim your life by improving your quality of life and reducing the numbers of symptoms, medications, and costs associated with Anxiety.

As we have, and continue to do, these general therapy recommendations must be tailored specifically to you the individual patient. Therefore, the recommendations herein are not "one size fits all." They must be considered by your physician specifically for you in light of your individual medical and personal history. Please do not consider any statement in this book as a diagnosis or prescribed therapy plan. These are guidelines to help educate. Again, THE INFORMATION IN THIS BOOK MUST BE CONSIDERED BY A PHYSICIAN AND APPLIED BY A PHYSICIAN BASED ON YOUR CLINICAL HISTORY.

Yes, there are pharmaceuticals recommended, and yes, we understand that many of you have been medicated "to death" and, as a result, no longer tolerate many medications that we may recommend. However, please understand that the dosages of pharmaceuticals are very low, and in most cases, homeopathic. Plus, the pharmaceuticals are recommended to help accelerate the relief that is usually brought about by the supplements and lifestyle modifications.

We hope that the information contained herein will restore hope for a better life and faith in the healthcare system, to enable you

Continued on page 5 . . .

Content Format

We include information to enable the physician to provide:

- Thorough clinical assessments,
- Patient education upon diagnosis,
- Assistance with interpreting and understanding the results of P&S monitoring, and
- Possible therapy options, including short-term, long-term, and lifelong.

The primary basis for this book is the science text: DePace NL and Colombo J. *Clinical Autonomic and Mitochondrial Disorders—Diagnosis, Prevention, and Treatment for Mind-Body Wellness.* Springer Science + Business Media, New York, NY, 2019.

For a more in-depth discussion on P&S monitoring consider the science text: Colombo J, Arora RR, DePace NL, Vinik AI. *Clinical Autonomic Dysfunction: Measurement, Indications, Therapies, and Outcomes.* Springer Science + Business Media, New York, NY, 2014. This book focuses on the science of fatigue in a less formal style.

Enjoy!

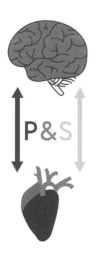

to work with your physician toward wellness. While not everyone, we have indeed helped most patients become active again and return to being a contributor to society. This is not to say that you may not need therapy lifelong. In fact, some do. However, the therapy may not require pharmaceuticals.

We include information to educate the patient so that they may help their physician and achieve health and wellness. To this end, we explain:

- How the P&S branches of the autonomic nervous system should work together in balance,
- How Dysautonomia (P&S imbalance) contributes to your symptoms of Anxiety,
- Why you may not have been properly diagnosed in the past,
- The clinical differences between Anxiety and Anxiety-like disorders,
- What to expect in working with your physician, and
- How to help.

Be Well!

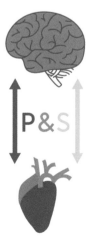

INTRODUCTION

Our first book in this series is about fatigue, both chronic fatigue syndrome and what we call persistent fatigue. Persistent fatigue refers to all those who are complaining of fatigue that do not fit the definition of chronic fatigue syndrome. We wrote about fatigue first because, in our experience, fatigue is the most commonly complained-about symptom. However, in our experience, Anxiety or rather (as we will define) Anxiety-like disorder is the most commonly diagnosed disorder. Like persistent fatigue, anxiety-like disorders are those patients who report symptoms of anxiety but do not fit the definition of anxiety. In fact, there is evidence that diagnoses of anxiety, including what we call anxiety-like disorders, are the most diagnosed condition worldwide—more diagnosed than heart disease and diabetes combined [1].

Background

The Strict Definition of Anxiety

The American Psychiatric Association (APA) classifies many psychological disorders under the umbrella of Anxiety. The classification that most people think of as "Anxiety" is Generalized Anxiety Disorder (GAD). From the APA's Diagnostic and Statistical Manual of Mental Disorders, Fifth Edition (DSM-5, 2013), the clinical definition of GAD is:

A. Excessive anxiety and worry (apprehensive expectation), occurring more days than not for at least six months, about a number of events or activities (such as work or school performance).

B. The individual finds it difficult to control the worry.

C. The anxiety and worry are associated with three (or more) of the following six symptoms (with at least some symptoms having been present for more days than not for the past six months): Note: Only one item is required for children.

D. The anxiety, worry, or physical symptoms cause clinically significant distress or impairment in social, occupational, or other important areas of functioning.
1. Restlessness, feeling keyed-up or on edge.
2. Being easily fatigued.
3. Difficulty concentrating or mind going blank.
4. Irritability.
5. Muscle tension.
6. Sleep disturbance (difficulty falling or staying asleep, or restless, unsatisfying sleep).

E. The disturbance is not attributable to the physiological effects of a substance (e.g., a drug of abuse or a medication) or another medical condition (e.g., hyperthyroidism).

F. The disturbance is not better explained by another medical disorder (e.g., anxiety or worry about having panic attacks in Panic Disorder, negative evaluation in Social Anxiety Disorder [Social Phobia], contamination or other obsessions in obsessive-compulsive disorder, separation from attachment figures in Separation Anxiety Disorder, reminders of traumatic events in Post-Traumatic Stress Disorder, gaining weight in Anorexia Nervosa, physical complaints in Somatic Symptom Disorder, perceived appearance flaws in Body Dysmorphic Disorder, having a serious illness in Illness Anxiety Disorder, or the content of delusional beliefs in Schizophrenia or Delusional Disorder).

The DMS-5 is the APA's text listing and describing all of the current recognized psychiatric disorders. In addition to GAD, they include Social Anxiety Disorder, Selective Mutism in Children, Panic Disorder, Agoraphobia and other Specific Phobias, Separation Anxiety Disorder, and Illness Anxiety Disorder. In the most recent definition of Anxiety disorders, the APA removed Post-Traumatic Stress Disorder and obsessive-compulsive disorder and listed them on their own, along with other related disorders. Attention Deficit

Disorder, Attention Deficit and Hyperactivity Disorder, Bipolar Disorder and other Depression-Anxiety disorders, and Manic Disorders, including Manic/Depression Disorder, are all known to also involve "anxiety."

YOU MAY NOT FIT THE STRICT DEFINITION.

THERE ARE MANY PATIENTS THAT DO NOT FIT THESE SPECIFIC CRITERIA.

THIS MAY BE YOU!

Based on the first book in this Mind-Body Wellness series *(FATIGUE & Dysautonomia: Chronic or Persistent, What's the Difference? The Mind-Body Wellness Program,* Skyhorse, 2023), we generalize "Item C.2. (Fatigue)" to include both chronic fatigue, as in chronic fatigue syndrome (CFS), and "persistent" fatigue, as in all the other fatigue patients that do not fit the specific APA criteria. Also, we generalize "Item C.3. (Difficulty concentrating or mind going blank)" to include "brain fog," difficulty finding words, as well as cognitive and memory difficulties typically associated with fatigue and the Dysautonomias that are associated with fatigue.

It may not be all in your head.

Anxiety disorders, and disorders having anxiety-laden symptoms as part of their presentation (what we will term "Anxiety-like" Disorders), affect millions of Americans at any given time, and many millions worldwide, and the numbers are growing rapidly. Anxiety, regardless of its form, may be more of a healthcare issue than people are willing to realize, and the effects are more insidious and pernicious. Anxiety disorders cause significant interpersonal, occupational, and economic burdens for the patients afflicted; and the family, friends and loved ones of those patients; and society as a whole, including businesses, schools, and governments. Given the fear-mongering of the news media, weather reporters, advertisers, and even the government, any form of anxiety will amplify the fear and subsequent responses to the cause of fear. This serves to increase depression and the risk of addiction (including obsessions for gaming and virtual reality devices, in addition to alcohol and drugs) and suicide as escape mechanisms. The need to escape or the feelings of depression are exacerbated if the individual feels there is no hope for a better future, including that which may be provided through a belief system.

Patients experiencing what is generally termed Anxiety may not actually have a psychological disorder. It may not be all in your head! Anxiety-like symptoms may be caused by physical symptoms (e.g., Dysautonomias) that lead to their primary Anxiety or Anxiety-like Disorder(s). That is right—as you will learn, not all symptoms or diagnoses of Anxiety are caused by mental health issues. The mental health, or psychologic, issue may be secondary to, or caused by, a physiologic health issue. This is the basis of the title to this book. Again, in these cases, *it may not be all in your head.*

Especially if medicated for more than three months . . .

Furthermore, a significant number of patients experiencing depression (whether clinical or preclinical) also have comorbid, or accompanying, symptoms of anxiety. Herein lies a clue. If patients diagnosed with Anxiety, or Depression-Anxiety syndromes (including Bipolar Disorder), have been on medications such as antidepressants or anxiolytics for more than three months (especially high doses of these medications) and still have bouts of anxiety or depression, there may be additional problems, or the problem may not be psychological at all. It may be what is known as a "brain perfusion" problem, known as brain hypoperfusion. That is a problem in your body that results in your brain not receiving enough (oxygenated) blood.

. . . or dehydrated.

A leading cause of brain hypoperfusion is dehydration. It may not be overstating the fact that approximately 40 percent of our patients are simply dehydrated. Given the predilection for caffeine, alcohol, and sugary drinks (including artificial sugars which may turn to alcohol in the blood), patients are fooled into thinking they are drinking enough. However, caffeine, alcohol, and sugar all dehydrate, which may also raise blood pressure, in which case, a common therapy is a diuretic which will further dehydrate. Remember, approximately 60 percent of your body is water, and you lose about half a gallon a day just from sleeping and normal activities, more if you are active. This needs to be replaced daily. If you also drink caffeine, alcohol, and sugary drinks, you need to add the same amount more water by volume of those other drinks to compensate, and then 48 ounces to 64 ounces in addition to remain properly hydrated. This may help to relieve some symptoms of anxiety, as well as depression and even hypertension (double-check with your physician in the hypertension cases). For women, proper daily hydration helps to keep skin and hair more supple and manageable. For those who do not like the taste of water or it makes them feel sick, it may be that their stomach (which is at a temperature of around 98°F) is contracting when colder water is drunk (even room-temperature water, which is around 70°F), pushing the stomach juices back up causing the bad taste or sick feeling. Sipping hot water (around 100°F, like from the tap) may resolve this issue; remember hot coffee or hot tea are just flavored hot water. Eliminate the caffeine flavoring and rehydrate.

With proper daily hydration, you increase your blood volume, reduce your blood viscosity, help your heart pump blood to the body, including the brain, and help to reduce anxiety and many other symptoms, as we will discuss.

Your brain may not be receiving enough blood.

When your brain is hypoperfused (under perfused or not receiving enough oxygenated blood), the first response is for your brain to signal an "adrenaline storm." This is meant to increase heart rate or blood pressure and open blood vessels and increase breathing, all to have more oxygenated blood sent up from the heart. Manifestations of this may include feelings of:

- **Restlessness**, where you want to exercise or do some physical activity to get blood flowing (circulating—your muscles help your heart to pump blood against gravity up to the brain); or
- **Irritability or emotionalism** of some sort, which are types of "psychological exercise" to increase circulation;
- **Shortness of breath**, to make you breathe more to bring in more oxygen and increase blood oxygenation; or
- **Palpitations and chest tightness or pain** (a feeling of a heart attack) due to the feeling of not pumping enough oxygen to the whole body, let alone the brain, or the feeling of increased pumping (like when exercising) even though you are at rest.

All of these symptoms are being caused to avoid the consequences of hypoperfusion. It does not necessarily mean you are having a heart attack. Yes, we understand those symptoms are scary. And, YES, *if you feel like you are having a heart attack, you should immediately seek medical attention and have those feelings checked*. But, PLEASE believe your doctors if and when they tell you that you are not having a heart attack. Emergency rooms are all filled with Anxiety or Anxiety-like patients who are not having a heart attack, but refuse to leave because they do not believe it. Granted, these symptoms exacerbate the perception of a heart attack, and perception is reality (for the patient), but test results (especially an EKG) do not lie, and the difference between a heart attack and not is very clear. So, please believe your doctors, calm down, and the symptoms will go away. In these cases, oftentimes, it only takes some proper hydration (like drinking some water) to relieve the symptoms of anxiety. Again, drinking a glass of water increases blood volume and boosts the sympathetics a little, both of which will help to deliver more blood to the brain, stopping the adrenaline storm, and relieving the anxiety-like symptoms.

Oftentimes, proper hydration
(like drinking some water)
relieves the symptoms of anxiety.

Brain hypoperfusion (not enough oxygenated blood to the brain) eventually results in the brain "going to sleep" and causing fatigue, malaise, brain fog, light-headedness,[a] confusion, memory and cognitive difficulties, difficulty finding words, and possibly gastrointestinal (GI) upset, headache or migraine, muscle pain in the neck and shoulders (what is known as "coat-hanger" pain), as well as other

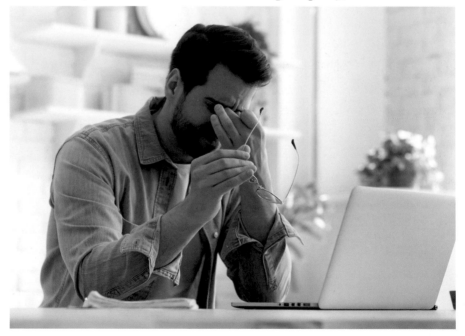

---

a In medical terminology, there is a difference between dizziness and light-headedness. While both seem to cause similar symptoms, medicine associates dizziness with Vestibular disorders and light-headedness with all other disorders, including Dysautonomias. With poor blood flow to the brain, since the Vestibular apparatuses are in your head, it is not uncommon to experience both. That is why doctors often mention both. They are not being redundant; they are being inclusive.

possible, less-common symptoms (e.g., muscle weakness, tremors or shaking, vision changes, dizziness, ringing in the ears, odd tastes or smells, strange feelings in the face or tongue, etc.). Not enough blood to the brain also means that there is not enough blood going to everything above the heart and possibly the heart itself.

Without sufficient amounts of blood, the brain is half asleep and a bout of depression is often the result and is often accompanied by the symptoms listed above and more: near-fainting or frank fainting (known as syncope) and more severe GI upset (including GERD, or persistent nausea or frequent vomiting). This is only one of several manifestations of the fact that the "problem is not all in your head." Other clues may include sleep difficulties, panic attacks, sex dysfunction, attention difficulties (including diagnoses of Attention Deficit Disorder [ADD], Attention Deficit and Hyperactivity Disorder [ADHD], obsessive-compulsive disorder [OCD]), eating disorders, or headache or migraine. These symptoms may also be a result of concussion or brain trauma and more. Brain trauma may include physical or mental trauma, including Post-Traumatic Stress Disorder (PTSD). These will be discussed later.

The Problem in Society

The psychiatry and psychology world is overwhelmed.

Over 70 percent of patients attempting suicide have at least one Anxiety disorder [2]. Local hospitals report up to twenty emergency room visits a day from patients having anxiety or panic attacks. Worse, up to half of these patients refuse to leave because they cannot believe that they are not having a heart attack or stroke. I have had personal friends, who are also patients, show up on my doorstep telling me they are having a heart attack when they were having a panic attack, and stay until the attack was over, even after several different attempts (including exams and tests) to prove to them that they were not having a heart attack. These societal problems are amplified by the fact that, currently, newly diagnosed Anxiety disorder patients may have to wait for up to six months to see a qualified psychiatrist. Given the growing numbers of patients with Anxiety disorder symptoms, the psychiatry and psychology world is overwhelmed. The sad truth of it all is that, according to some reports, up to 12 percent of these patients are lost to suicide during these six months.

12 percent are lost to suicide
(circa. 2020).

The problem is compounded by the fact that, by some estimates, there is currently (circa, 2020) a need for over 10,000 psychiatrists, but less than 2,000 are scheduled to be licensed in the near future. People need help, and the traditional source of help is simply not available. Nontraditional sources of help must become more well-known and available. This is another motivation for writing this book. If it is demonstrated that the cause of your anxiety may not be "all in your head," there are other causes that may be treated and relieved by non-Psychiatrists. Then at least some of the physiological symptoms related to Anxiety are reduced, thereby reducing your Anxiety and helping you and your psychiatrist to focus on the true mental health issue, if one persists.

We Have Two Brains

Nontraditional sources of help, including P&S monitoring,
must become more well-known and available.

Another way to consider this is the fact that you actually have two brains in your body: the one in your head and one in your "gut." The "Gut-Brain" is a well accepted concept, but is not well-known because it is hard to measure and monitor. Relatively very little of this "Gut-Brain" is actually taught in medical schools, because there is very little data. The "Gut-Brain" includes portions of your

Autonomic Nervous System (ANS), including its two branches: the Parasympathetic and Sympathetic (P&S) nervous systems. A reason why the P&S systems are hard to measure is because they are "hidden" behind your organs. They control and coordinate your organs. In fact, they control or coordinate virtually every cell in your body, including your brain, your heart, your immune system, your stomach, everything. The P&S nervous systems connect your brain, your heart, and your mind to your body.

As one simple example, the P&S nervous systems are the cause of the "butterflies" in your stomach before you must present yourself to people, such as in a performance or when you are to meet the special person on whom you are sweet. The emotion or stress created in the mind causes the brain to want to empty the stomach in case you need to fight or flee, to "lighten the load" as it were. Now the technology exists to measure and monitor the P&S nervous systems: P&S monitoring. Now the data are available to your physician which provide more information to relieve the suffering, improve quality of life (reduce morbidity risk), and reduce the rate of associated life-threatening conditions and suicides (mortality risk) that often result from Anxiety and Anxiety-like disorders and other Dysautonomias.

Psychosocial Stress

Psychosocial stress is arguably the major cause of diseases and disorders worldwide. Given the Mind-Body connection, mental stress increases and prolongs Sympathetic activity, which is supposed to only be reactionary (short-term). This results in a prolonged "fight or flight" condition, amplifying the stress and resultant symptoms of anxiety. Prolonged Sympathetic activity causes systemic changes (increases in heart rate, blood pressure, insulin levels, inflammation, histaminergic reactions, etc.), which is not only damaging to systems, it is damaging to the very cells that form those systems. Stress at the cellular level is known as oxidative stress. Like prolonged psychosocial stress, prolonged oxidative stress (in the cells, like the apple in the insert below, left) interferes with cell function and cell structure and, perhaps most significantly, cellular energy production by damaging the mitochondria (the power plants of cells), reducing the production of the "energy molecule" ATP [3]. This is the top of the slippery slope and the beginning of the cascade of symptoms that typically present, secondary to Anxiety or Anxiety-like disorders.

For example, society seems intent on causing Anxiety at every turn. Girls, from the day they first watch television, or see a popular magazine, are visually assaulted with the "perfect female form." Typically, it is a form that is impossible for girls to live up to—even the girls in the pictures themselves, as these pictures are made "perfect" with computer technologies: blemishes are "air-brushed" away, breasts and hips are augmented, tummies are tightened, and faces are modified slightly all with computers to sell the perfect image. This is compounded by the lack of a father or trusted father figure in so many families. In the young girls' lives, their fathers are supposed to be their first and best "boyfriend." This absolutely **does not** include any sexual actions. It does include **proper** touching, including **proper** hugging. More specifically, it also includes building up his daughter's self-esteem, self-awareness, self-confidence, and self-image. The simple compliment of "You look pretty" from the father does more to dispel the daughter's self-doubt as she tries to compare herself to the world's images that she is plagued with, than anything else in her life, including the same compliment from Mom. Dad is the first and most powerful male figure in a young girl's life. If she does not receive that healthy love from her father or trusted father figure, she will seek it elsewhere, and it is all too often not healthy, and that search only serves to deepen her anxiety and depression.

Girls are not the only victims of society's attacks. More boys are raped by authoritative women in their lives than society is willing to admit, or they are forced to engage in sexual contact with men, including the male figures in their lives they are supposed to look up to, model, and imitate. This situation is not helped by the fractured family unit, the very group of people which are the sources of a boy's self-esteem, self-awareness, self-confidence, and self-image. The self-doubt in boys is deepened by society's concept of the perfect male, one that is self-dependent and independent, one that is not emotional or "weak"—just "suck it up and deal" is the direction from society. Without the emotional release in a safe environment, boys internalize these issues, and too often the result is depression and anxiety. Both gender issues are more confused now by society's blurring of the identities associated with each.

Safe Haven Lost

The news is another significant source of anxiety for all. No news is good news. The news seems to be all about death tolls (in fact, the news media seems to go out of their way to find disasters that caused death), including murders, shootings, stabbings, abuse, abandonment, war, terrorism, weather disasters, and the like. In this, the media exports psychosocial stress to the common person. The media brings the ultimate fear (death) into the living rooms and bedrooms of all. Yes, we need to care that people are harmed in such a way, and we realize that the "world is shrinking," but when the "local" news reports on these sorts of things from hundreds or thousands of miles away, it is no longer local, and impacts the sense of security we all need for mental and physical health. The effect of the media and the immediacy and availability of this bad news through the ubiquitous display screen (television, computer, tablet, cell phone, etc.) has called into question these once safe and secure places of home, school, and church or temple; places of security.

As mentioned, another, formerly safe and secure place is also now questioned: schools. These safe places are being further invaded by Hollywood's obsession with death, including the undead (zombies and vampires). It is a curious fact that the children of the top management of the companies that provide some type of technology that is on or in your television, computer, tablet, or cell phone, go to private schools that refuse admission of any electronic device. In fact, they only use actual blackboards and chalk, and "force" the student to read actual books (with real paper) that are found in a physical library with a paper based card catalogue, and write with actual ink (or graphite) on paper and carry notebooks; meanwhile, the rest of the world is living and learning through the screen or monitor. Furthermore, these private-school students are being "forced" to use their *own* imaginations!

Churches, Synagogues, and Mosques are also questionable safe havens. These places are meant to speak hope into peoples' lives, yet due to bigotry, hate crimes, and the general lack of tolerance toward different people, these places of hope have also been threatened and invaded. Without hope, anxiety has no bounds.

Borrowed Imagination

Using one's own imagination is a skill that has been lost on many in the younger generations. Through television, movies, video games, and now virtual reality, they are borrowing others' imagination and creativity. This has impacted society in the reduction of new inventions and innovations, even in the reduction of new movies. Fewer books are read (even if electronically) and more are "reading" a book by watching the movie made from the book (and never actually reading the book, but saying that they have). For example, I read the series of books by JRR Tolkien on the Hobbits. Tolkien has an incredible style of writing that fires the imagination and seems to bring you directly into the realm he creates, stimulating all of the senses (new sights and sounds, new languages, etc.). Then I saw the movies. I hated the movies! That is at first, because nothing looked or sounded right. Nothing looked or sounded like I had imagined it. They looked and sounded like what someone else imagined, what the creators of the movie imagined. I was being forced to accept their imagination. This fact made it worse. Today's children are not reading as much and are filling their time (or having their time filled—the smartphone has become the new baby-sitter) with images and "virtual reality" that are developed from someone else's imagination and creativity, and we wonder why our society has lost that creative and innovative leadership in the world?

Moral Compass Lost

Ultimately, society has lost its moral compass. Man (as in humans) has become the standard. Unfortunately, this is a bad standard; it is too low. For once some woman or man reaches that standard, the standard must be raised. In other words, the standard is a moving target which simply frustrates society; it is no longer a standard. A result (especially in the government) is that the standards become so low that they are no longer standards. This is done so that no one is left out, but then where is the motivation to excel and improve one's self? For example, there was a time when the criterion to receive an award was to outperform *all* others. Now all children receive awards for simply participating or even just showing up. What, you think the children do not know the score? Through some religions, perfection and the infinite (as defined by that religion) is the standard—something unattainable by any mortal. Therefore, we (mortals) were all in the same boat. We were all imperfect, and as such could relate better with each other, working with each other to cover our imperfections and accentuate our perfections. This is the basis of a good marriage and a healthy family. While there are valid reasons for divorce (e.g., mental or physical abuse), the lack of a desire to work together is not a good reason and is the reason for the high divorce rate and the depression-anxiety complexes that divorce causes, especially in the children—no matter what their age.

If this is not you or yours, great;
keep up the good work!

The point is that without helping your child develop her/his own imagination, self-esteem, self-awareness, self-confidence, and self-image, s/he will become a teenager who cannot imagine what they want to be, and they will never "find themselves." As a result, they will be depressed and anxious for life. You can help by "unplugging" your child/children for a couple of hours a day. You may even get them to exercise during that time (more than their thumbs, by running and old-fashioned play), as well further increase the health of our population. You may also help them to learn how to communicate, face-to-face, using their mouth (and not their thumbs). It will be one less class they will need to take (and you will need to pay for) in college, if they get there. Yes, colleges are now including communication courses as part of the core (required) curriculum. These classes teach etiquette and how to interact with others, person-to-person, without any electronics; this is something that the older generations learned at home.

Of course, proper nutrition, from a proper diet, and exercise are key factors. Without proper diet and exercise, healthy blood flow and coronary (heart) and brain perfusion and many other functions may be compromised, and anxiety is promoted. The Western lifestyle, with stress (including psychosocial stress) and a diet of convenience (a diet that is "fresh from the factory," not "farm" fresh), is significantly contributing to anxiety as well. The lack of good nutrition and healthy exercise exacerbates anxiety and depression (by increasing oxidative stress, among other things), including anxiety due to fear of, or presence of, illness.

"Keeping up with the Joneses" is an impossible task. Society highlights the very few that are so rich that the common person is never happy with what they have, nor is satisfied with living within their means. Worse, for those who do get something extra, there is always someone else who has more to "have" to live up to.

The family is being shredded. This includes all the confusion around sexual identity, the rampant divorce rate, and the alarming abortion rate. Again, humans are the standard; this makes life cheap, including babies and fetuses. If women want control over their bodies, exercise it before getting pregnant! True, there are extreme circumstances, but they account for an extremely low percentage of the reasons for abortion. Note, no matter how strong the woman, the hormonal, emotional, and chemical changes that occur in a women's body due to abortion are never lost. They have permanent effects on mental and physical health and are life changing.

Technology has only helped to further the family-shredding. All people, including very young children barely weaned, are now bombarded with images most adults should never see, as well as being isolated by the video screen and are not taught how to interact with people. From deafness research (deafness is the most isolating of all sensory deficits), a deaf person in a group with no other deaf people around becomes isolated, withdrawn, and, on average, has a significantly shorter life expectancy; perhaps up to 30 years shorter. This is attributed to the lack of social interaction.

Humans are made to be in community, in relationship. Among the other things listed, community helps to grow and strengthen our immune systems. Our first immunity (typically) comes from our mother at birth (vaginal birth). Then it is grown through vaccinations and play. Playing (especially outside, in the sunshine—which has many important benefits, both mentally and physically) is very important in the growth of the immune system as the children (think of them as "germ-sponges") crawl all over each other and eat their pound of dirt each day. Even adults touch (shake hands, hug, kiss, etc.) and share germs with each other. All of this makes us stronger (assuming you are not at risk). Isolation, including behind a video screen, is not healthy. All of these excesses need to be balanced, just like a foundation of health is a balance between the Parasympathetic and Syathetic branches of the Autonomic Nervous System.

Ultimately all of this is underscored by the lack of a universal standard. The religions of the world used to help people be happy and secure with what they are endowed, and they teach community. Now they have become prosperity religions, or the basis to try to make everyone conform to themselves. There is no comfort, no concern, especially for others. "Do unto others as you have them do unto you" has become "Do unto others before they do unto you." No universal standard means that there is no standard. First of all, standards set by people are too low. This is why, secondly, the standards are always changing. For once the standard is

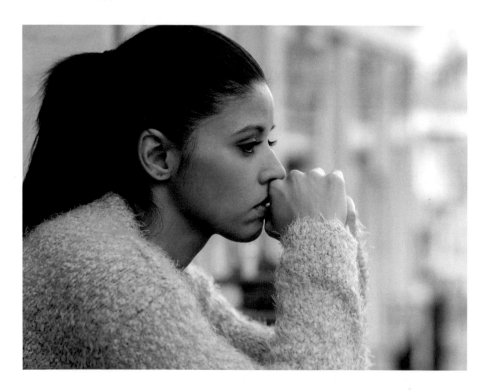

met by someone, people will raise the standard to prove they are the best. Of course, the governments lower the standards so that everyone may conform. All of this provides absolutely no security and leads to rampant anxiety. However, a standard of perfection with love enables everyone to do their best, working together to accentuate their strengths, and living happily with the results. That is more security and less anxiety: "the Peace that surpasses all understanding."

To review, Anxiety disorders often include several physiologic symptoms, including: sleep difficulties, GI upset, heart palpitations, high blood pressure or difficult to control blood pressure, elevated or high heart rate, abnormal sweating, light-headedness, and experiences of depersonalization and derealization. These physiologic symptoms all involve the Parasympathetic and Sympathetic nervous systems (P&S). In fact, it is possible that this combination indicates that there are abnormalities (including excesses) in both systems [4]. Stress plays a significant role in the pathology of Anxiety disorders [5]. Stress includes psychosocial stress at the systemic level and growing evidence of oxidative stress at the cellular level [6,7,8,9,10]. Oxidative stress significantly affects the P&S and is associated with autonomic disorders such as neurogenic orthostatic hypotension[b] [11]. Orthostatic dysfunction is arguably one of the most debilitating of autonomic disorders [12,13]. The physiologic symptoms, above, plus light-headedness, cognitive and memory difficulties, "Brain Fog," sex dysfunction, shortness of breath, and persistent fatigue (not necessarily chronic fatigue syndrome) from orthostatic dysfunction help to define Anxiety or Anxiety-like-Disorder, (collectively referred to as "Anxiety-like") symptoms.

---

b Neurogenic orthostatic hypotension (NOH) is diagnosed based on tilt- or postural change study when a patient demonstrates a 20/10 mmHg drop in BP from rest to upright posture. NOH is a diagnosis. In general, orthostatic dysfunction references the symptomatology of the various orthostatic disorders: NOH, orthostatic hypotension, postural orthostatic tachycardia syndrome and orthostatic intolerance.

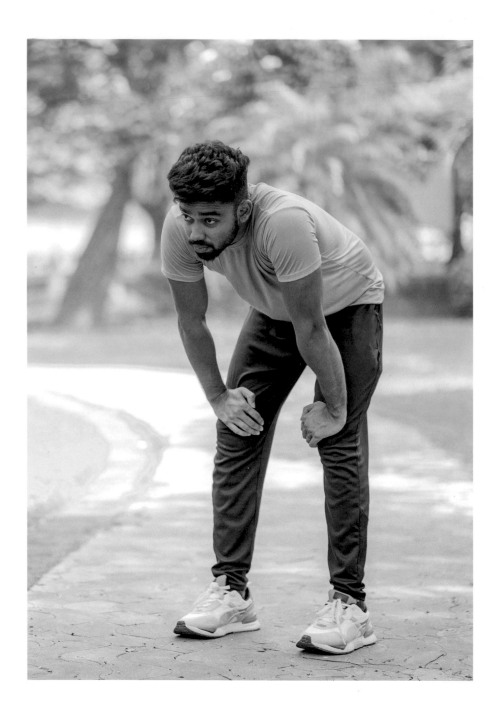

MIND-BODY WELLNESS PROGRAM BASICS

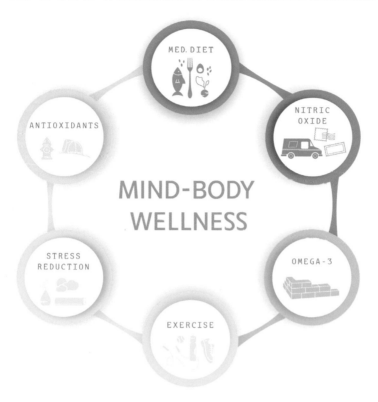

The brain and the heart are key to WELLNESS. They are connected to each other, and the rest of the body, by the Parasympathetic and Sympathetic (P&S) nervous systems and blood (via the vasculature). These systems control and coordinate all the other systems. Keeping these systems healthy and WELL helps to maintain WELLNESS throughout the rest of the systems of the body, and thereby maximizes quality of life (by minimizing morbidity risk) and maximizes longevity (by minimizing mortality risk).

Quality of life, as defined for an adult, would include:
- eating and sleeping well,
- regular bathroom habits,
- having sex,
- normal blood pressure, and
- not getting dizzy or fatigued frequently.

The Mind-Body Wellness Program is designed to provide you maximum quality of life and longevity. It does so by recommending its "Six prongs to WELLNESS:"

1. **Omega-3 Fatty Acids** are the membrane molecule. They provide the building blocks for our membranes, like the stones in a stone wall (as in the insert, right). However, unlike stones, omega-3 fatty acids also help to keep cell walls supple and receptive (represented by the flowers) to passing into the cell the raw materials necessary to support WELLNESS as well as passing out those which do not.

2. **Nitric Oxide** is the anti-atherosclerotic molecule. With a supporting cast of **amino acids, vitamins, and minerals** it keeps the body operating as a WELL-oiled machine. It is a policeman, regulating blood flow and preventing traffic jams (clots). It is a fireman preventing inFLAMmation that causes white blood cells to adhere to blood vessel walls. It is a paramedic, repairing membranes throughout the body. It is an engineer, building new blood vessels (roads) to efficiently supply the entire body. It is also an antioxidant.

3. **Antioxidants** (**Alpha Lipoic Acid** and **CoQ10**, the body's own "super-antioxidants") are used to prevent stress at the cellular level from both inflammation and oxidative stress (oxidation is burning—a fire is an oxidation reaction), including keeping the immune system and the power plants of the body—the mitochondria–WELL. In fact, antioxidants support the health of all systems throughout the body, and help to keep them healthy, energized, and WELL. There are two forms of Alpha-Lipoic

Acid (ALA), r-ALA and s-ALA. Only r-ALA is active in humans, s-ALA is often used as filler in supplements that state a "proprietary blend of ALA" to help keep costs down. Unfortunately s-ALA is not active in humans and makes little differnce to your wellness.

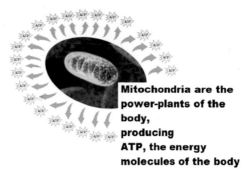

Mitochondria are the power-plants of the body, producing ATP, the energy molecules of the body

The three lifestyle prongs (following) of the **Mind-Body Wellness Program** all provide antioxidant protection. In fact, exercise may just be the most potent of all antioxidant processes. These two particular antioxidants are the most powerful, natural antioxidants we have. Your body produces them. Not only are they the most powerful in and of themselves, they make themselves even more powerful by recycling other antioxidants, like vitamins A, C, and E. Without r-ALA and CoQ10, these vitamins typically make only one pass through the body. Note, the reason why the literature has so many differing opinions on the efficacy and dosing of these vitamins as antioxidants is because most experiments (assuming they were actually performed) did not account for the level of ALA or CoQ10. ALA and CoQ10 are both produced in the human body, and that production decreases with age and duration of chronic disease.

4. **Mediterranean Diet** is a lifestyle to fuel our bodies with the ingredients required for WELLNESS, while avoiding ingredients that promote the diseases of our time that are becoming epidemic (over fifteen types of cancer, dementia, atherosclerosis, and diabetes). It includes eating mostly whole grains, fruits, and vegetables. The protein is obtained from eating mostly fish and seafood, lean meats, eggs, cheese, yogurt, and milk. It includes very little processed fats and sugars. The lifestyle aspect is that it mostly includes fresh, in-season, unprocessed foods: "factory fresh" (as in fresh from nature) not "fresh from the factory." The other lifestyle aspect is the way food is consumed. It should be consumed in a relaxed environment, at a table, with friends and family laughing and talking together. All of this good food and good company may be aided by a small glass of wine.

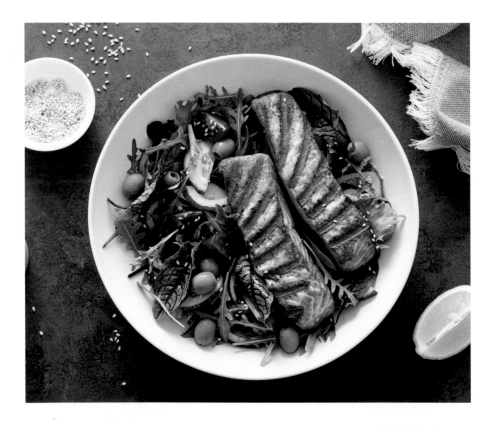

5. **Exercise.** *It is not a dirty word!* It is a fountain of youth lifestyle for WELLNESS. Think of it in terms of an active lifestyle, the lifestyle that preceded automobiles, elevators, television remotes, and cell phones. Examples include common housework, gardening, walking, and taking the stairs. It does not have to include going to the gym or beating yourself up to feel good. In fact, if you only feel good while exercising and feel more pain and fatigue after exercise, you may be exercising too hard and your body may be perceiving that level of exercise as a stress, albeit a healthy stress. We are not discouraging those who do workout harder, and benefit from it and enjoy it, but it is not the minimum requirement. The recommended minimum is 150 minutes of moderate exercise per week. Perhaps a little more for young children.

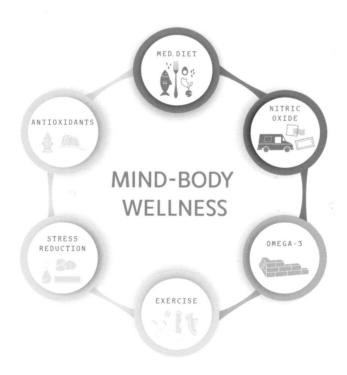

6. <u>Psychosocial Stress Reduction</u> is a lifestyle to prevent stress at the system level, promoting a happy, *"laughter is the best medicine,"* kind of WELLNESS.

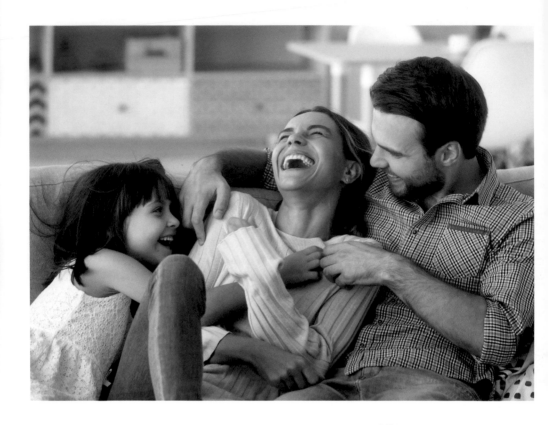

The Mediterranean diet and exercise work together to provide the foundations for health and WELLNESS. Exercise and psychosocial stress reduction help to keep the body happy, reducing pain and inflammation, and enabling you to enjoy your health and WELLNESS!

All SIX PRONGS are important and are to be taken together as a whole.

PARASYMPATHETIC AND SYMPATHETIC (P&S) MONITORING

Parasympathetic and Sympathetic (P&S) monitoring provides more information, helping to improve differential diagnoses and therapy planning. This more information may also help to identify disease and disorder earlier, even before symptoms present. P&S monitoring goes beyond customized medicine, promoting "individualized" medicine. As a result, it may reduce medication load, hospitalization and re-hospitalization, reduce morbidity and mortality risk, improve patient outcomes, and thereby reduce healthcare costs. Morbidity risks directly affect quality of life, and mortality risks directly affect length of life. Establishing and maintaining P&S balance goes a long way toward BEING WELL.

The P&S Nervous Systems

The Parasympathetic Nervous System is commonly referred to as the "rest and digest" nervous system. It is responsible for conserving energy and establishing metabolic baselines. In many situations, it acts like the brakes on a car. It is the "protective" nervous system. The Sympathetic Nervous System is commonly referred to as the "fight or flight" nervous system. It is responsible for expending energy. In many situations, it acts like the accelerator on a car. It is the "reactionary" nervous system. The ANS is one of the main human systems responsible for Man's capability and adaptability. The interplay between the P&S branches underlies this ability; they also form the communication network between the mind and the body, including the brain and the heart.

The P&S nervous systems' responses collectively constitute an individual patient's physiologic "fingerprint." It may provide more information to help to reduce medication load (assuming

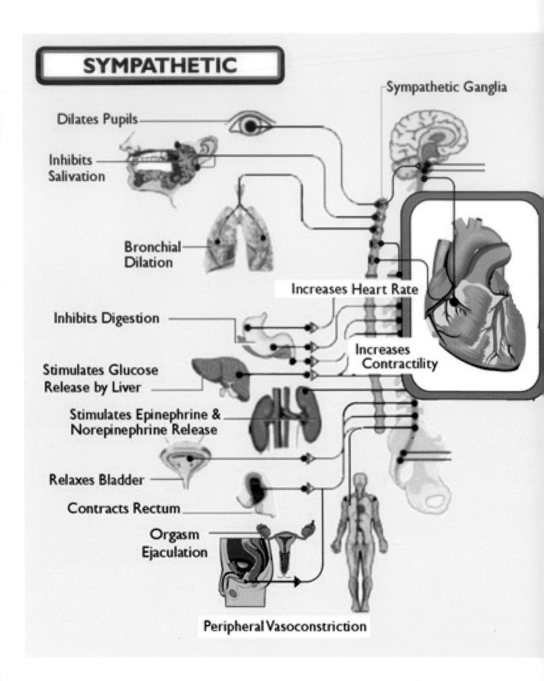

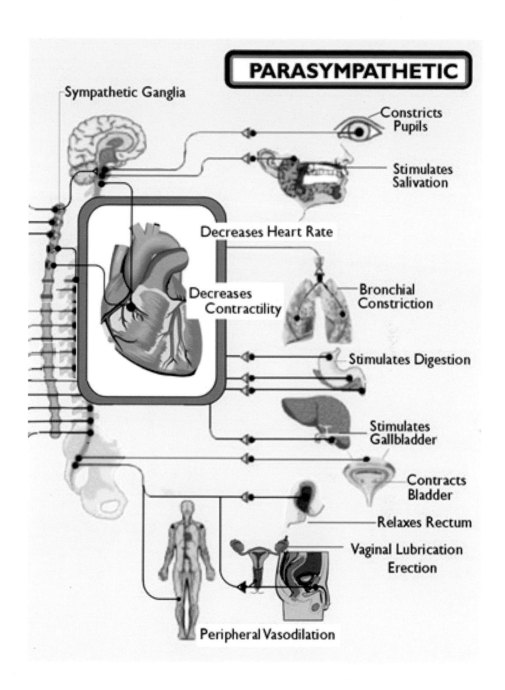

no end organ effects) by providing more information about the underlying disease state or disorder. The previous page displays some of the functions of the P&S Nervous systems. A typical chronic disease patient, whose symptoms are being treated one at a time, may be prescribed three agents for high blood pressure, two medications for GI symptoms, two medications for sleep disorder, and one or more medications for Anxiety; and may still have a poor quality of life. All of these symptoms (perhaps due to Anxiety, for example) may be due to a Parasympathetic dysfunction with a Sympathetic dysfunction. Symptoms of Parasympathetic dysfunction may include GI symptoms, sleep disorders, and any underlying depression.

Symptoms of Sympathetic dysfunction may include hypertension or high blood pressure. In cases of Anxiety, in addition to treating all of the above symptoms, individually, with medication, anxiolytics may be prescribed for the Anxiety and probably beta-blockers for the palpitations that accompany Anxiety. However, oftentimes, P&S monitoring documents this a primary Parasympathetic condition with the Sympathetic symptoms secondary. Unfortunately, it is often treated as a Primary Sympathetic condition and at best barely manages the whole. As a primary Parasympathetic condition, it may be treated with one medication and a low-dose medication at that. Relieving Parasympathetic dysfunction may relieve all of the Parasympathetic-related symptoms with the one medication. Then, by relieving the Parasympathetic dysfunction, (eventually) the Sympathetic dysfunction and its related symptoms will be relieved. Once Parasympathetic dysfunction is relieved, the patient may not need to stay on the medication (again, assuming no end organ effects), for the nervous system learns and by this method may be "retrained" to maintain a new and healthier balance.

Continuing the Anxiety example, many Anxiety patients believe they are having a heart attack and visit the emergency room (ER).

After testing, many patients still refuse to believe they are not having a heart attack and will not leave the ER. These patients continue to feel shortness of breath, chest tightness, and palpitations. However, if these symptoms are demonstrated to not be from a heart attack, then they are often a result of the "adrenaline storm" produced by the brain to call for more oxygenated blood. The shortness of breath feeling is to make you breathe more to increase blood oxygenation. The chest tightness and palpitations are the body's responses to the increase in adrenaline that is spurring on the increase in blood pressure and heart rate (respectively) to increase blood flow to the brain. Not only do extended ER stays consume resources unnecessarily, but they also include unnecessary transportation costs. Remote P&S monitoring avoids all of these costs, helping to keep the patient at home.

To review, as you know, the Parasympathetic and Sympathetic (P&S) branches of the ANS work synergistically to control and coordinate the function of all bodily systems and virtually every cell in the body. The Sympathetics are the "fight or flight" system. They are the reactionary system. Sympathetic responses are meant to be short in duration (relative to the Parasympathetics), working in the acute phase of systemic responses to stresses (whether healthy or not). They react to the physiologic, or metabolic, threshold set by the Parasympathetics.

"Brakes" & "Accelerator"

To further develop a useful analogy, the Sympathetics are like the accelerator of a car. In many instances, they accelerate functions of the body. Yet they are the slower of the two branches to respond. As in a car, you never want the accelerator working faster than the brakes, or you may not be able to stop the car and may crash. In the body, examples of the "crash" are a heart attack or a stroke. The majority of the Sympathetic nervous system outside the brain arises from the Sympathetic Chain ganglia just outside the spine (see previous figure). There are other components to it as well, including the Angiotensin-Renin-Aldosterone system. Of course the adrenal glands, including adrenaline and cortisol, are significant factors that influence and are influenced by the Sympathetics. The Sympathetics uniquely control the vasculature. The most common manifestations of Sympathetic responses are changes in HR & BP, as well as histaminergic and other inflammatory responses.

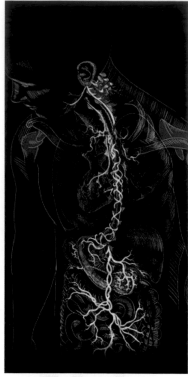

The Vagus Nerve

The Parasympathetics are the "rest and digest" system. As mentioned, they set the metabolic and physiologic thresholds around which the Sympathetics react in any given situation. Parasympathetic responses are meant to be more chronic, although protracted Parasympathetic responses are also unhealthy, as in brain injury (concussion or trauma) or some conditions thought to be autoimmune. The most common effects of protracted Parasympathetic activity are depression and fatigue.

The Parasympathetics are the protective branch of the ANS, ensuring proper tissue perfusion throughout the body (for physicians who remember from medical school: that is why long Valsalva maneuvers are very strong Parasympathetic stimuli, and short Valsalva maneuvers are powerful Sympathetic stimuli). When the body has been insulted too often or too traumatically, the Parasympathetics may remain activated for too long, causing many diffuse, seemingly unrelated, symptoms, and it may cause the patient to be difficult to manage, especially regarding

BP, blood sugars, hormones, and weight. The majority of the Parasympathetic nervous system outside the brain is the Vagus Nerve (see previous figure above for functions, also the **insert left** for an indication of its anatomy). Of course, there are also Sacral, Nitrergic, and Enteric nerves that also carry Parasympathetic information outside the brain. The pathways that are Parasympathetic inside the brain are throughout the brain (Cerebrum, Midbrain, and Brain stem), including (1) the brain stem ganglia that house the cell body's that give rise to the Vagus Nerve, (2) related ganglia that deal with the body's reward system, (3) the Limbic system, and (4) hormonal systems. Outside the brain, the Parasympathetics uniquely control the GI tract. The most common manifestations of Parasympathetic responses are Respiratory Sinus arrhythmia (the only arrhythmia you want) and gastric motility ("butterflies in the stomach" in response to stress).

P&S balance directly affects morbidity and mortality risks, including quality of life. Adult quality of life may be defined as eating and sleeping well, proper bowel and bladder function, proper sex function, and normal BP and orthostatic responses. All of these are controlled or coordinated by the P&S nervous systems.

To continue developing our analogy, the Parasympathetics would be like the "brakes" of the body. Under normal conditions, for common activities, the following analogy describes the interaction between the P&S systems, the brakes and accelerator, respectively. As in a car (with an automatic transmission), if you are at a red light with your foot on the brakes and the light turns green, what is the first thing you do? . . . You take your foot off the brakes. . . . Even before you touch the accelerator, you begin to roll, you already begin to accelerate. Taking your foot off the brakes minimizes the amount of gas (read that as adrenaline) and acceleration (read that as Sympathetic stress) you need to reach your desired speed. The P&S nervous systems normally act in much the same manner: 1)

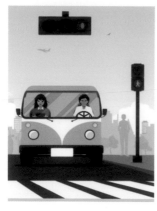

first the Parasympathetics decrease to facilitate and minimize the Sympathetic response, and 2) then a small Sympathetics increase to sustain the Sympathetic response.

Note, the car analogy does not exclude the "seesaw" model of the ANS taught in medical school. According to the "seesaw" model, normally, when one branch is active (high), the other branch is not active (low, see figures to the right). However, this occurs mostly in healthy subjects, and significantly less often in patients. The "seesaw" model is inherent in the "brake and accelerator" model. Normally, when one's foot is on the gas, there is not a foot on the brakes, and vice versa. The benefit of the "brake and accelerator" model is that is goes further in explaining many abnormal conditions, for example, Parasympathetic Excess with Sympathetic Excess (the autonomic dysfunction most associated with Depression-Anxiety syndromes; see the "broken" seesaw figure).

In the "seesaw" model, the "seesaw" is broken, but there is no extension of the analogy. In the "brake and accelerator" model, this is like driving a car with a foot on the brakes and accelerator at the same time. This helps to explain the situation much more fully, as you will see.

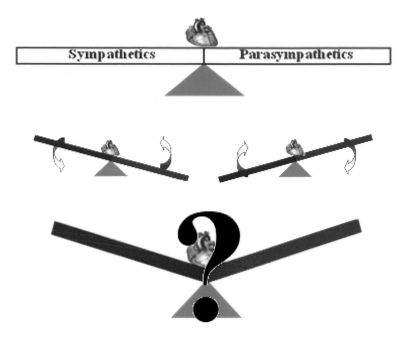

Autonomic Dysfunction

A failure of the proper interaction between the P&S leads to disorder and possibly disease. To extend the analogy, if you do not take your foot off the brakes and hit the accelerator, you still go, but you must use much more gas (again, read that as "adrenaline") and you must over-rev your engine (read that as "over stimulate the Sympathetics" or overstress yourself) to go anywhere. This places more wear on the engine (the heart, kidneys, and body) and on the brakes (the Parasympathetics). A problem is, in the human, once the "brakes" (the Parasympathetics) wear out, they cannot be replaced. Even without an accelerator, eventually you will roll down a hill and crash; that may be the heart attack, stroke, fatal electrical arrhythmia, or severe orthostatic intolerance with chronic fatigue.

In clinical terms, "no brakes" is known as Cardiovascular Autonomic Neuropathy (CAN), and is associated with increased mortality risk (risk of life-threatening illness or death). While this is normal for older geriatrics (after all, the risk of a normal eighty-five-year-old dying is higher than that for a normal forty-five-year-old) or patients with long-term chronic illness, it becomes clinically significant (and should be treated) if CAN presents with a resting P&S balance (known as Sympathovagal Balance or SB[c]) greater than 2.5. In clinical terms, CAN with high SB indicates that your Parasympathetics are not strong enough to prevent a sympathetically mediated Ventricular Tachy-rhythm from becoming fibrillation that may lead to a heart attack or stroke. Therefore, to prevent the "brakes" (the Parasympathetics) from wearing out too fast, the recommended therapy is based on "getting your foot off the brakes" (reducing Parasympathetic activity) to minimize wear on the "brakes" and thereby the "engine." This may include anticholinergic therapy, also known as very low dose antidepressant therapy, on the order of $1/10^{th}$ the traditional dose of antidepressants.

"Over-revving your engine," which is exaggerating or overstimulating stress responses, is Sympathetic Excess (SE) and may be a primary Dysautonomia or secondary to Parasympathetic Excess (PE). SE secondary to PE is like riding the brakes while driving the accelerator. In these two types of cases (primary SE or SE secondary to PE), the beta-sympathetics are being overstimulated. Beta-sympathetics mediate heart and lung function. There is another sympathetic dysfunction which involves an alpha-sympathetic insufficiency known as Sympathetic Withdrawal (SW, not hitting the accelerator at the red light and rolling backward; the blood stays in the feet and ankles rather than being moved to the heart). The alpha-Sympatheics mediate vascular tone. SW indicates a condition where the lower vasculature does not help to return blood to the heart, which makes the heart work harder to pump blood to the

---

c SB = (resting Sympathetic activity)/(resting Parasympathetic activity), Normal range: 0.4 < SB < 3.0;

Preferred normal for geriatric and chronically ill: 0.4 < SB < 1.0;

Preferred normal for younger patients: 1.0 < SB < 3.0;

brain. These three Dysautonomias (SW, PE, and SE) may explain the symptoms of:

- Anxiety: where small worries are amplified and large worries may become mentally crippling;
  - SW or PE may cause reduced blood flow to the brain (reduced brain perfusion pressure) and when the blood pressure in the brain drops further due to some other event, the brain issues an "adrenaline storm" which may cycle Anxiety-like symptoms; or
  - PE may induce secondary SE, and the SE may simulate an "adrenaline storm," which again may cycle Anxiety-like symptoms;
  - SW, PE, and SE may all occur together, compounding and complicating the condition.
- Pain Syndromes: where normal stimuli (light touch and tickle) are amplified into pain responses and significant pain response may become physically crippling;
  - Fibromyalgia: this may also be associated with generalized, widespread pain such as in Fibromyalgia, where the pain is due to poor tissue perfusion due to the "brakes" (the Parasympathetics) limiting the ability to pump more blood under stress—"acting as a governor on the engine." This may contribute to "coat-hanger" pain, or pain in the shoulders and neck area[d], however SW seems to be the primary cause of "coat-hanger" pain. In fact, any area above the heart (including the brain and perhaps the heart itself) is not receiving enough blood due to PE or SW, and therefore pain results, including chest pain. This may also include headache, often mistaken as tension headaches, especially those that are not relieved by common analgesics;

---

d The primary cause of "coat-hanger" pain symptoms is Sympathetic Withdrawal (SW, which we will discuss later). SW is the neurological basis of orthostatic disorders. It is the abnormal Sympathetic response to postural change where the Sympathetics decrease rather than increase.

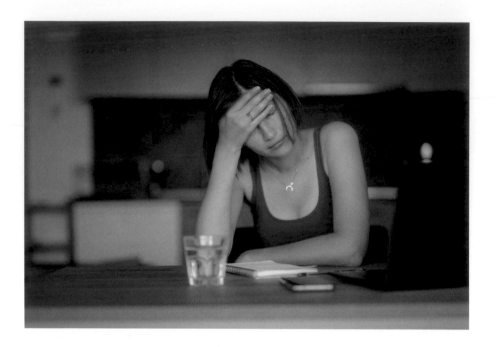

○ Chronic Regional Pain Syndrome (CRPS, not differentiated): is basically the combination of the above two conditions: 1) "normal" (somatosensory) pain, involving SE, as a result of the injury, and 2) "pins and needles" type pain due to poor tissue perfusion to the affected area(s), involving PE causing reduced blood flow to that area. In this case PE is a response to the compromised vascular supply to the area resulting from the injury (e.g., a crushed plexus), and the Parasympathetics are seeking a solution to the reduced tissue perfusion.

Hitting the "brakes" or "riding the brakes" explains the symptoms of:

• Addiction: Again, consider you are driving your car. As you are driving and everything is normal and calm, suddenly something unexpected occurs. What is your first reaction? . . . You hit the brakes. Again, your body is very similar. The "brakes" (the Parasympathetics) are the protective mechanism. In addiction, the "brakes" cause the patient to seek their "comfort zone," whether it be drugs, alcohol, sex, food, or whatever is their compulsion. The Parasympathetics are strongly associated with the "Pleasure Centers" or "Comfort Centers" of the brain stem. Once addicted, the Parasympathetics tend to remain excessive. If the Parasympathetic Excess is not relieved during rehabilitation, then the risk of relapse remains high due to the excessive (Parasympathetic) drive in the patient to remain in their "comfort zone" stimulating their "pleasure centers;"

- "Brain Fog" and Cognitive and Memory Difficulties: PE and SW contribute by: (PE) limiting the output of the heart under stress, or (SW) shifting blood volume away from the heart. Either and both result in poor brain perfusion, which results in reduced brain activity, similar to that associated with depression.

- Fatigue: Often patients describe their symptoms as if they were "running a marathon while sitting still." PE will cause this by causing normal responses to little, normal stresses to be amplified into excessive responses, increasing cardiac function, metabolism, and energy expenditure while doing little if anything. SW contributes to fatigue by shifting blood volume away from the heart, resulting in poor brain perfusion, which results in reduced brain activity ("Sleepy Brain"), similar to that associated with depression.

- Sleep Difficulties: If you take more than 20 minutes to fall asleep, or wake more than twice a night (even to go to the bathroom), then your sleep difficulty may be caused by PE or SW, both of which limit blood flow to the brain. Consider what happens when a patient faints. Besides gravity working, once flat on the ground, the heart and head are at the same level. Their brains are receiving all the blood it wants; it's happy, the patient is not. Similarly, after being upright all day (sitting or standing), as soon as the patient lies down to go to sleep, their brain (which has been partially asleep all day) now has all the blood it wants; it wants to play, the patient wants to sleep (the patient typically lays there processing their day, reviewing lists of things to do, and planning for the morrow). In restoring proper brain perfusion (blood flow to the brain), the brain will wake up, process the day, and then, with the normal brain changes with evening, the brain will be ready for sleep when the patient is.

The Thermostat Analogy

As you know, the first symptom of sudden cardiac death is often death itself. Similarly with stroke, stroke is the first symptom. P&S monitoring when applied early may detect these mortality risks early. CAN with high P&S Balance (high SB) is associated with a 50 percent increase in the two-year mortality rate in chronic heart disease patients and patients with diseases that place them at risk for heart disease, including diabetes and COPD. Given that the definition of CAN is very low, resting, Parasympathetic activity, like worn-out brakes on a car, unfortunately the "brakes" in the human system cannot be replaced. Perhaps a better analogy for sudden death and stroke and other mortality risks (including MACE) is a **thermostat** and the associated cooling and heating systems (Parasympathetic and Sympathetic systems, respectively).

Assume you have no knowledge of, nor are able to see, hear, or access the cooling and heating systems of your house. All you have to assess the function of those systems is the thermostat on the wall. Say you set the temperature on the thermostat to 70°F (like 70 beats per minute for heart rate). Assume it is a hot, humid summer day. Assume that the cooling system is healthy. Now assume that a $5.00 heater switch fails and the heater turns on to full capacity. What happens to the temperature of the house as measured by the thermostat? . . . *NOTHING!* . . . The cooling system amps up to compensate not only for the ambient heat but also for the heat from the heating system. Now both systems are operating at full capacity, and the thermostat temperature still reads 70°F, and everyone is still happy. However, how long will this situation last until there is a catastrophic failure in one or both of the air conditioning systems? Only after a catastrophic failure does the temperature change. Then it is too late, and the repair is $5,000.00 or more. The change in temperature, indicating a failure, is too late! The $5.00 repair is simpler, and easier, but you have to be measuring both the cooling and heating systems, not just the net result of their combined activities.

The Autonomic Nervous System in the human body is very similar in this regard. We are still surprised by heart attacks and strokes, and other organ failures, because we only measure total ANS function (the net result of the P&S nervous systems) and not the individual P&S nervous systems themselves. This is made more poignant by the fact that it is the purpose of the P&S nervous systems to work together to maintain normal organ function, even when they themselves are dysfunctional (like the heating and cooling systems

"Thermostat Analogy"

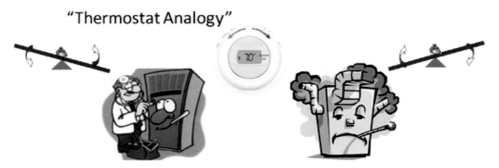

P&S maintains normal organ function even when the
P&S themselves are abnormal

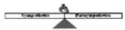

maintaining 70°F in failure mode). Current, common place health-care measurements are made more effective and efficient with the additional information of P&S monitoring.[e]

P&S monitoring provides more information. It is the only non-invasive technology that quantifies Parasympathetic activity, independent of, and simultaneously with, Sympathetic activity. All other noninvasive autonomic technologies force assumption and approximation to theorize P&S activity. P&S monitoring technology was developed in animal models through the 1980s with chemical, electrical, and mechanical blockade studies [14,15,16,17]. By the early 1990s, P&S monitoring was verified and validated in humans. Both the animal and early human studies were performed at MIT and Harvard medical school. The majority of the human studies were performed at beta-sites throughout the US, including Harvard, Cleveland Clinic, Univ. of Pennsylvania, Stanford University, and fourteen others. P&S monitoring was USFDA cleared in 1995 and US Medicare accepted in 1997. It continues to be patented and well-published in numerous journals of many clinical disciplines.

To briefly summarize, P&S nervous systems are "hidden" behind the organs and control and coordinate them, providing more and possibly earlier information to aid in diagnosing and treating chronic disease. Independent, simultaneous measures of P&S (dys)function is not otherwise available. Typically, by the time symptoms present, the disease or disorder is well progressed, and therapy is often lifelong. More information, earlier, reduces the need for lifelong therapy.

---

e   With other autonomic tests, even if their assumptions and approximations are correct, they are not measuring the separate activities of the two branches at the same time. For instance, first they measure P-activity against deep breathing, then they measure S-activity against Valsalva. They cannot measure the direct interactions between the two branches to the same stimulus.

The terms SE, PE, and SW will be formally introduced and detailed in the body of the text. To extend the car analogy, SE is like "over-revving your engine" which is exaggerating or overstimulating your stress responses (Sympathetic responses). PE is like "riding the brakes." Often, PE causes SE, but the SE in these cases is virtually always secondary to the PE and must be treated as such so as to not exacerbate both Dysautonomias.

The Mind-Body Connection

The P&S nervous systems are the brain-heart, or more generally, the mind-body connection. P&S monitoring is more information about the physiologic condition of the individual patient. It also has ramifications regarding the mental health of the individual as well, as it provides data regarding brain perfusion and sleep function. Typically, if a patient is monitored early, the P&S information is earlier than other physiologic measures. Remember, the P&S nervous systems control the organs, and its purpose is to maintain normal organ function even when it, itself, is abnormal. Ultimately, abnormal P&S function will be translated to the organ system or systems. As an aside, this is why there is usually an onset latency to post-trauma syndromes, for example, or autonomic dysfunction in pre-diabetes 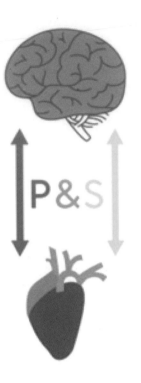 or even metabolic syndrome, long before diabetes is diagnosed. Also, given that the P&S nervous systems are the repositories of the individual patient's health history, including the memory for the immune system (which is why vaccines are helpful), we may state that P&S monitoring documents the patient's individual and specific "physiologic fingerprint."

P&S monitoring provides more information to healthcare providers throughout the fields of healthcare and beyond, including chronic care, critical care, mental health, assisted living (including nursing homes), and for wellness programs. The more information helps providers to reduce morbidity and mortality risk, and reduce medication load, and therefore reduce hospitalization and re-hospitalization, all the while improving patient outcomes and reducing costs.

P&S monitoring independently and simultaneously quantifies both autonomic systems. As recently published, all other noninvasive, autonomic, single, beat-to-beat cardiac measures are not sufficient to characterize P&S activity [18]. With P&S monitoring, it is not necessary to default to invasive neural testing to get more precise quantitative data in more benign autonomic dysfunction situations, especially if it is not a life-threatening condition. All other noninvasive autonomic measures are based on only the one beat-to-beat measure of the heart and therefore are only a measure of total autonomic function. The other autonomic measures are, therefore, ambiguous and force assumption and approximation to theorize P&S activity.

P&S monitoring provides more information for chronic care medicine, which typically is the majority of national healthcare costs. P&S-guided therapy often relieves multiple symptoms at the same time, rather than only treating the individual symptoms in isolation. Furthermore, if there are no end organ deficits, P&S-guided therapy is often not lifelong. In these cases, it is possible to "retrain" the P&S systems (like breaking a bad habit and establishing and stabilizing a good habit). Once stabilized, the P&S systems may carry forward on their own without the help of therapy until some other clinical event occurs. To this end, if a condition is detected early enough, before symptoms, P&S therapy is preventative and short-term (usually nine to eighteen months).

Ultimately, chronic disease, like Anxiety, accelerates the onset of autonomic dysfunction, including Cardiovascular Autonomic Neuropathy (CAN, defined as very low, resting Parasympathetic activity and is late- to end- stage autonomic dysfunction). In summary, P&S-guided therapy reduces morbidity and mortality risks, reduces medication load, improves patient outcomes, and reduces costs.

The Clinical P&S Test

To test the P&S nervous systems, a multi-phased test is necessary, primarily due to the fact that the P&S systems are dynamic systems. Most medical tests are not dynamic; patients are at rest (sitting or supine) when tested. The P&S nervous systems are never resting. Even when you are asleep, the nervous system is active, arguably more active than when you are awake. Therefore, typically, patients are tested, diagnosed, and treated to normalize their resting state. Unfortunately, most P&S disorders are not demonstrated while at rest. Therefore, a dynamic test must be administered. Another need for a dynamic P&S test is that a patient is seen only periodically by a physician. Information representing the patient's responses when not in the physician's office helps to better manage the patient. However, it is also helpful to be able to diagnose and initiate therapy on the first test.

The resulting test is a fifteen-minute, thirty-five-second test (see next figures, page after next):

A. The first five minutes is a resting baseline that enables the patient to become their own control, enabling same-day diagnosis and therapy.

B. Deep or Paced Breathing at six breaths per minute for a minute. Six breaths per minute is the average optimal stimulus for the human Parasympathetic nervous system. Deep Breathing simulates patient responses to disease and therapy after large meals, before bedtime, and other Parasympathetic dominant situations.

C. The patient is then returned to baseline and normal breathing for a minute.

D. The Valsalva challenge is five short Valsalva maneuvers, with intervening rest periods over a minute and thirty-five seconds. Valsalva maneuvers simulate patient responses to disease and therapy during stress, exercise, and other Sympathetic dominant situations. This includes the standard fifteen-second Valsalva and helps to document baroreceptor reflex function.

E. The patient is then returned to baseline and normal breathing for two minutes.

F. The last five minutes include a quick change from sitting to standing or tilt. Either way, it is a head-up postural change challenge. In fact, this portion of the test largely replaces a tilt test [19]. The stand challenge is important for documenting the causes of light-headedness, as discussed in the hypertension example. It is also important for documenting the coordination between the P&S nervous systems. If they do not coordinate properly (as in the "break and accelerator" analogy) for something as common as standing, they may not be coordinating the organs properly. Which organ is significantly affected is determined based on symptoms or further testing as needed, given the patient's medical history.

If the patient uses a wheelchair and cannot stand for even a couple of minutes, then the entire test may be performed supine and the patient either quickly tilted (if on a tilt table) and remain tilted for the five minutes, or requested to quickly sit up and remain with proper seated posture for the five minutes.

None of these challenges should cause symptoms. While the patient should not talk during the test, if there are symptoms, even if they are mild, the patient should let the technician know immediately. The reason is that symptoms may be more revealing than borderline results. To this end, the test is still valid even if the patient cannot complete some of the challenges. If symptoms are significant, then abort the challenge and, if needed, reseat the patient and finish the challenge, then continue the rest of the test.

Introduction

To minimize artifact, there should also be no moving during the test, unless otherwise directed.

Unless directed by your physician, do not change or alter your therapy protocol or your typical lifestyle. It takes the nervous system up to three months to fully adapt to a change in therapy or lifestyle. Therefore, a short-term (one- or two-day) change will not have a significant effect.

Please avoid a significant meal within half an hour of testing or a significant exercise period within an hour of testing. In this case, significant exercise may include climbing a flight of stairs if the patient has heart failure, for example.

The test will require you to have three EKG electrodes placed on your chest and a blood pressure cuff placed on your arm. For comfort and convenience, wear a two-piece outfit, with no body lotions, oils, or sprays.

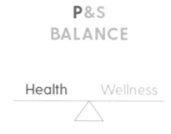

TESTING PROCEDURE

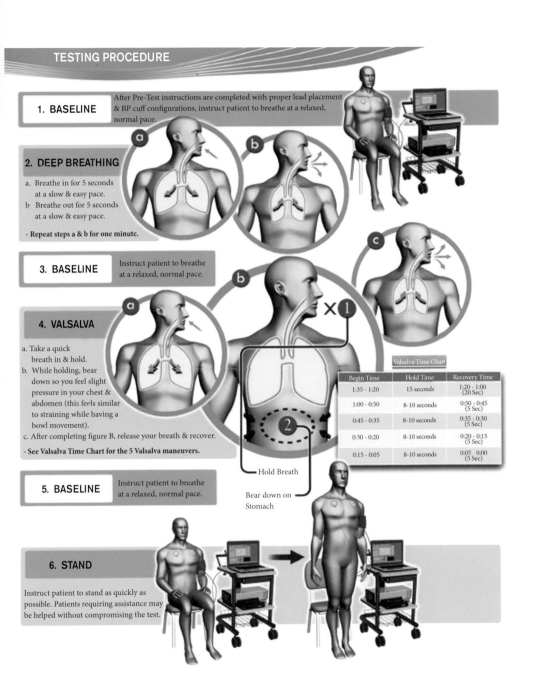

1. BASELINE

After Pre-Test instructions are completed with proper lead placement & BP cuff configurations, instruct patient to breathe at a relaxed, normal pace.

2. DEEP BREATHING

a. Breathe in for 5 seconds at a slow & easy pace.
b. Breathe out for 5 seconds at a slow & easy pace.

- **Repeat steps a & b for one minute.**

3. BASELINE

Instruct patient to breathe at a relaxed, normal pace.

4. VALSALVA

a. Take a quick breath in & hold.
b. While holding, bear down so you feel slight pressure in your chest & abdomen (this feels similar to straining while having a bowl movement).
c. After completing figure B, release your breath & recover.

- **See Valsalva Time Chart for the 5 Valsalva maneuvers.**

Hold Breath

Bear down on Stomach

Valsalva Time Chart

Begin Time	Hold Time	Recovery Time
1:35 - 1:20	15 seconds	1:20 - 1:00 (20 Sec)
1:00 - 0:50	8-10 seconds	0:50 - 0:45 (5 Sec)
0:45 - 0:35	8-10 seconds	0:35 - 0:30 (5 Sec)
0:30 - 0:20	8-10 seconds	0:20 - 0:15 (5 Sec)
0:15 - 0:05	8-10 seconds	0:05 - 0:00 (5 Sec)

5. BASELINE

Instruct patient to breathe at a relaxed, normal pace.

6. STAND

Instruct patient to stand as quickly as possible. Patients requiring assistance may be helped without compromising the test.

DISCLAIMERS

Mr. Parker has no conflicts of interest.

Drs. DePace and Colombo are the authors of the book upon which this is based:

DePace NL, Colombo J.
Autonomic and Mitochondrial Dysfunction in Clinical Diseases: Diagnostic,
Prevention, and Therapy.
Springer Science + Business Media, New York, NY, 2019.

While we have developed the supplement package described as part of the Mind-Body Wellness Program, all of these supplements are readily available through common commercial means (i.e., your neighborhood pharmacy). Only at the insistence of our patients have we packaged the supplements for sale as a convenience.

Drs. DePace and Colombo are some of the authors of the book upon which the implementation and application of P&S monitoring is based:

Colombo J, Arora RR, DePace NL, Vinik AI.
Clinical Autonomic Dysfunction: Measurement, Indications, Therapies, and
Outcomes. Springer Science + Business Media, New York, NY, 2014.

Drs. DePace and Colombo are co-owners of the research organization from which some of the data included herein was collected and analyzed: NeuroCardiology Research Corporation.

Dr. Colombo is a co-owner, Chief Technology Officer, and Senior Medical Director of Physio PS, Inc., the producer and provider of P&S monitoring technologies.

The information and contents, including medical information, in this book are solely and strictly offered as an educational and informational resource. The use of this book shall be expressly limited as an informational tool to help improve awareness and understanding of Dysautonomia in Anxiety and Anxiety-like syndromes for both patients and physicians. This book is not intended to, and does not claim to, provide any medical or professional advice or diagnosis, or medical or professional opinion, or medical or professional treatment services of any kind, whether pharmaceutical, supplemental, nutraceutical, or lifestyle, to any individual. This book shall in no way substitute or replace the patient-physician relationship or be used as a substitute for medical or professional diagnosis and treatment. Please consult a board-certified physician for medical advice or treatment and before making any decisions or changes in your healthcare treatment plan(s).

We wish all a lifetime of happiness and wellness.
Enjoy!

P&S
BALANCE

Health   Wellness

ANXIETY SYMPTOMS

ATTENTION DISORDERS
COLD CHILLS
BRAIN ZAPS
WORRY
MEMORY LOSS
CONFUSION
MANY THOUGHTS
SHORT OF BREATH
DEPERSONALIZATION
BRAIN FOG
RINGING IN THE EARS
EYE STRAIN
TWITCHING
PRESSURE
WEAK
RACING HEART
DIFFICULTY
JUMPY
BLURRED VISION
BOLD JOLTS
WEIGHT LOSS
MUSCLE TENSION

DIFFICULTY FOCUSING
FALLING SENSATION
CHRONIC FATIGUE
LIGHT HEADED
HEADACHES
DIZZINESS
TREMBLING
FEELING LIKE PASSING OUT
WEIGHT GAIN
STOMACH PAIN
HOT FLASHES
PALPITATIONS
NIGHT SWEATS
SHAKING
NAUSEA
CHEST PAIN
RESTLESS LEGS
SWEATING

ANXIETY

HISTORY

First, here is a little history [20], then we start the physician-patient format. Da Costa syndrome or "A Soldier's Heart Syndrome," known also as "Soldier's Heart" or "Effort Syndrome," this phenomenon was another ailment commonly seen in World War I. Arthur Hurst stated that it "may be associated with prolonged mental strain and insufficient sleep, on a heart and nervous system weakened by the action of some form of Toxemia." Da Costa syndrome is named for the surgeon Jacob Mendes Da Costa [21], who first observed it in soldiers during the American Civil War. At the time it was proposed, Da Costa syndrome was seen as a very desirable physiological explanation for "Soldier's Heart" [22]. Use of the term "Da Costa syndrome" peaked in the early twentieth century. Toward the mid-century, the condition was generally re-characterized as a form of neurosis [23]. It was initially classified as "F45.3" (under Somatoform Disorder of the Heart and Cardiovascular System) in ICD-10 [24], and is now classified under "Somatoform Autonomic Dysfunction."

Da Costa syndrome involves a set of symptoms which include left-sided chest pains, palpitations, breathlessness (shortness of breath), sweating, and fatigue in response to exertion. Earl de Grey presented four reports on British soldiers with these symptoms between 1864 and 1868 and attributed them to the heavy weight of military equipment being carried in knapsacks which were tightly strapped to the chest in a manner which constricted the action of the heart. Also in 1864, Henry Harthorne observed soldiers in the American Civil War who had similar symptoms which were attributed to "long-continued overexertion, with deficiency of rest and often nourishment," and indefinite heart complaints were attributed to lack of sleep and bad food. In 1870, Arthur Bowen Myers of the Coldstream Guards also regarded the accoutrements as the cause of the trouble, which he called Neurocirculatory Asthenia and Cardiovascular Neurosis [25,26].

J. M. Da Costa's study of three hundred soldiers reported similar findings in 1871 and added that the condition often developed and persisted after a bout of fever or diarrhea. He also noted that the pulse was always greatly and rapidly influenced by position, such as stooping or reclining. A typical case involved a man who was on active duty for several months or more and contracted an annoying bout of diarrhea or fever, and then, after a short stay in hospital, returned to active service. The soldier soon found that he could not keep up with his comrades in the exertions of a soldier's life as previously, because he would get out of breath, would get dizzy, and have palpitations and pains in his chest, yet upon examination sometime later, he appeared generally healthy [27]. In 1876, surgeon Arthur Davy attributed the symptoms to military drill where "over-expanding the chest, caused dilatation of the heart, and so induced irritability" [25].

Since then, a variety of similar or partly similar conditions have been described. Da Costa syndrome is a syndrome with a set of symptoms that are similar to those of heart disease. While a physical examination does not reveal any gross physiological abnormalities, orthostatic intolerance has been noted. It was originally thought to be a heart condition, and treated with a predecessor to modern cardiac drugs. While the condition was eventually recategorized as psychiatric [28,29], in modern times, it is known to represent several disorders, some of which now have a known medical basis. It is also variously known as Cardiac Neurosis, Chronic Asthenia, Effort Syndrome, Functional Cardiovascular Disease, Primary Neurasthenia, Subacute Asthenia, and Irritable Heart [30,31,32,33]. None of these terms have widespread use.

The term Da Costa syndrome is no longer in common use by any medical agencies and has generally been superseded by more specific diagnoses, some of which have a medical basis. Although it is listed in the ICD-9 under "Somatoform Autonomic Dysfunction" [28], the term is no longer in common use by any medical agencies and has generally been superseded by more specific diagnoses.

The orthostatic intolerance observed by Da Costa has since also been found in patients diagnosed with chronic fatigue syndrome, postural orthostatic tachycardia syndrome (POTS) [34,35] and Mitral Valve Prolapse Syndrome [36]. In the twenty-first century, this intolerance is classified as a neurological condition. Exercise intolerance has since been found in many organic diseases.

The report of Da Costa shows that patients recovered from the more severe symptoms when removed from the strenuous activity or sustained lifestyle that caused them. A reclined position and forced bed rest was the most beneficial. Other treatments evident from the previous studies were improving physique and posture, appropriate levels of exercise where possible, wearing loose clothing about the waist, and avoiding postural changes such as stooping, or lying on the left or right side, or the back in some cases, which relieved some of the palpitations and chest pains, and standing up slowly can prevent the faintness associated with postural or orthostatic hypotension in some cases.

NOW TO THE MAIN BODY OF THE BOOK

in physician—patient format.

PHYSICIAN: ANXIETY AND DYSAUTONOMIA

Anxiety can become a pathologic disorder (1) when it is excessive and uncontrollable, (2) when it requires no specific external stimulus, (3) when it manifests with a wide range of physical and affective symptoms, and (4) when it is accompanied by changes in behavior and cognition. Patients often present with complaints of poor physical health as their primary concern. If only symptoms are considered, this can be misleading. Poor health is particularly common in Panic Attacks due to Anxiety, which are characterized by a short period of intense fear and a sense of impending doom, with accompanying physical symptoms, such as chest pain, light-headedness or dizziness, and shortness of breath. Very often, these patients first present to an emergency department (ED). Unfortunately, many of these patients refuse to leave the ED once they have been assured they are not having a heart attack, unnecessarily consuming healthcare resources due to the comorbid fear.

Anxiety is one of the most prevalent of all psychiatric disorders in the general population. Simple Phobia is the most common Anxiety disorder, with up to 49 percent of people reporting an unreasonably strong fear and 25 percent of those people meeting criteria for Simple Phobia. Social Anxiety Disorder is the next most common disorder of Anxiety, with roughly 13 percent of people reporting symptoms that meet the DSM criteria. PTSD, which is often unrecognized, afflicts approximately 7.8 percent of the overall population and 12 percent of women, in whom it is significantly more common. In victims of war trauma, PTSD prevalence reaches 20 percent [37], and probably more. A subjective experience of distress with accompanying disturbances of sleep, concentration, and social or occupational functioning are common symptoms in many of the Anxiety Disorders.

Despite their similarities, these disorders often differ in presentation, course, and treatment. Diagnosis is often complicated by other psychiatric and physiologic disorders.

PATIENT: ANXIETY AND DYSAUTONOMIA

Anxiety is a natural response and a necessary warning adaptation in humans. However, Anxiety is meant to be, like all Sympathetic responses to stresses, a temporary, transient reaction. It was never meant to be prolonged. Unfortunately, in the modern world, there are many stresses that are constant. For example, we were not designed to live in a world with a restaurant on every corner. Food has become a stress and a cause for Anxiety. Humans, while designed to be in community with other humans, were meant to be dispersed, not crowded together in dense populations. Although the world is not overcrowded, there are certain areas of it that are and that has led to many types of Anxiety, mostly from psychosocial stresses. Other societal psychosocial stresses are mentioned in the Introduction. Prolonged stress, resulting in prolonged Sympathetic activation, leads to poor health and often includes Anxiety, either or both, Primary or Anxiety-Like Disorders.

Anxiety may include Panic Attacks, obsessive-compulsive disorders, ADD/ADHD, PTSD (either or both mental or physical), Manic behaviors, Phobias, and Depression-Anxiety syndromes, including Bipolar Disorder. Poor health is often associated with Anxiety. Attacks often include a short period of intense fear and a sense of impending doom with accompanying physical symptoms, such as chest pain, light-headedness or dizziness, and shortness of breath.

Again, Anxiety is arguably the most commonly diagnosed disorder worldwide. Many of its symptoms are, themselves, potentially debilitating (e.g., persistent fatigue, malaise, exercise intolerance, fear, etc.) and often effect quality of life, the ability to work or function in society or in the family, and often places patients at increased morbidity and mortality risk, including increased risk of suicide or substance dependency.

In cases of Anxiety with P&S Dysfunction, or Dysautonomia,

Many Anxiety disorders have overlapping signs and symptoms, requiring the clinician to explore several lines of questioning to clarify the primary diagnosis. Anxiety disorders that are more commonly recognized have lower lifetime prevalence rates. GAD and Panic Disorder, for example, have lifetime prevalence rates of roughly 5 percent and 3.5 percent, respectively. Of the panic sufferers, up to 40 percent also meet criteria for Agoraphobia.

A significant concern of the psychiatrist is that, in many cases, the patient becomes fixated on the physiologic symptoms of Anxiety (sleep disorder, GI upset, sex dysfunction, fatigue, memory and cognitive difficulties), consuming much of the psychiatrist's time, without attending to the psychology of the Anxiety itself. P&S-guided therapy helps to relieve the physiologic symptoms, enabling more attention to the psychologic symptoms.

Clinically important risk factors leading to Anxiety and Anxiety-like disorders include comorbid substance abuse and family history (including possible genetic predisposition[f]). One twenty-year study of the offspring of depressed parents found a threefold increase in Anxiety disorders, including greater substance abuse, younger onset, and more significant physical health concerns [38]. Otherwise, definitive pathophysiologic mechanisms have not yet been determined for Primary Anxiety. However, Anxiety symptoms and the resulting disorders are believed to be due to disrupted modulation within the central nervous system, including: hormonal and neurotransmitter imbalances; trauma, stroke, and other brain injuries (including concussion); and poor brain perfusion.

---

f   There is also a possible genetic predisposition to autonomic dysfunction, including PE, which may underlie Anxiety.

relieving the P&S Dysfunction significantly reduces the impact of Anxiety, helping to restore quality of life, and the ability to work or function, reduces morbidity and mortality risk, often reducing medication load, hospitalizations and re-hospitalizations, and overall reducing healthcare costs for both the individual and society.

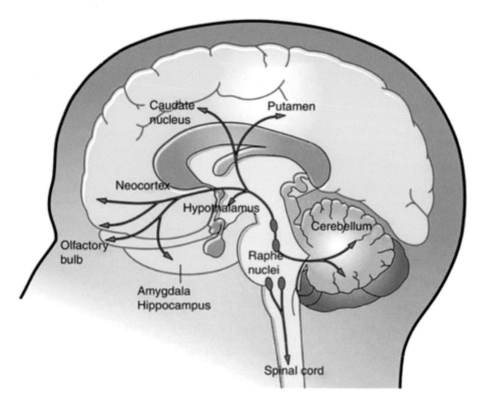

Figure 1: Serotonin is one the two most commonly considered neurotransmitter systems. Principal Serotonergic projections from the reticular formation are displayed [3]. Several of these main projections involve the P&S, especially the Amygdala. Also, serotonin is a major neurotransmitter in the gut and the "Gut Brain." [with permission, 133, Fig. 4,8]

Environmental stressors clearly play a role to varying degrees. All Primary Anxiety disorders are affected in some way by external

In primary Anxiety, the most commonly considered neurotransmitter systems are the serotoninergic (Figure 1) and Noradrenergic (Figure 2) systems. In very general terms, it is believed that an under-activation of the serotoninergic system and an over-activation of the Noradrenergic system are involved. These systems regulate and are regulated by other pathways and neuronal circuits in various regions of the brain, including the Locus Coeruleus and limbic structures, resulting in dysregulation of physiologic arousal and the emotional experience of this arousal, and the involvement of the P&S Nervous Systems, that also engage bodily systems.

Environmental stressors clearly play a role to varying degrees. All primary Anxiety disorders are affected in some way by external cues. Abnormal processing of, and responses to, these cues often underlie Primary Anxiety. Physical and emotional manifestations of this dysregulation are the result of heightened Sympathetic arousal of varying degrees; including SE secondary to PE (see p. 22). The Anxiety, worry, or physical symptoms cause clinically significant distress or impairment in social or occupational functioning. Several neurotransmitter systems have been implicated in one or several of the modulatory steps involved.

In some forms of Primary Anxiety, a disruption of the Gamma-Aminobutyric Acid (GABA) system has also been implicated because of the response of many of the Anxiety-spectrum disorders to treatment with Benzodiazepines. There has also been some interest in the role of Corticosteroid regulation and its relation to symptoms of fear and anxiety. Corticosteroids might increase or decrease the activity of certain neural pathways, affecting not only behavior under stress but also the brain's processing of fear-inducing stimuli.

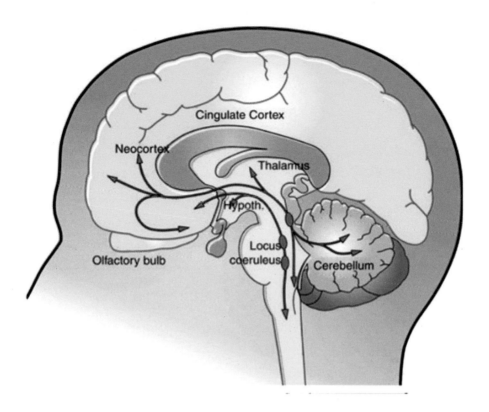

Figure 2: Noradrenaline or norepinephrine (they are the same chemical) is one of the two most commonly considered neurotransmitter systems. Principal Noradrenergic projections from the reticular formation are displayed [3]. Noradrenergic neurons are part of the Sympathetic nervous system and are influenced by the hormone, adrenaline, both inside the brain and throughout the body, including the "Gut Brain." [Figure, with permission, 133, Fig. 4.6]

cues. Abnormal processing of, and responses to, these cues often underlie Primary Anxiety. Physical and emotional manifestations of this dysregulation are the result of heightened Sympathetic arousal of varying degrees, including SE secondary to PE. The anxiety, worry, or physical symptoms cause clinically significant distress or impairment in social or occupational functioning. Several neurotransmitter systems have been implicated in one or several of the modulatory steps involved.

DEFINITIONS AND DIAGNOSTICS

Anxiety is a complex disorder that may not always be only psychological. We will differentiate two general types of Anxiety disorders: Primary Anxiety and Anxiety-like Disorders (ALD). The term "Anxiety" will refer to both types in general. ALDs, specifically those resulting from Dysautonomia(s), will be referred to as "P&S Anxiety." The strict definition of what we are calling Primary Anxiety is detailed in the Introduction. In summary, Primary Anxiety includes an number of subtype as defined by the APA (DSM-5, 2013): Generalized Anxiety Disorder (GAD), Social Anxiety Disorder (also known as Social Phobia), Specific Phobia, Panic Disorder with and without Agoraphobia, Post-Traumatic Stress Disorder (PTSD), Anxiety secondary to medical condition, Acute Stress Disorder (ASD), and Substance-Induced Anxiety Disorder [39]. Therefore, by definition, persistent psychosocial Stress is Anxiety. PTSD will be addressed separately in another book in this series; however, many of its issues parallel those of anxiety as discussed herein. PTSD tends to be more complex. The DSM-5 no longer includes obsessive-compulsive disorders as Anxiety. Through (physiological) work in the P&S nervous system, additional forms of "Anxiety" have been documented [40,41]; however, the only "Anxiety" that is officially recognized is (primary) Anxiety, which qualifies under the DSM-5 definition (e.g., Generalized Anxiety Disorder. 300.02 (F41.1) A, and its related forms, as listed above). In general, Anxiety is clinically defined as "excessive anxiety and worry (apprehensive expectation), occurring more days than not for at least six months, about a number of events or activities (such as work or school performance)" [39].

Many patients do not meet the criteria for any of the Primary Anxiety classifications, yet they feel Anxiety; they have anxiety-laden symptoms as part of their presentation. Recognizing that patients

DEFINITIONS AND DIAGNOSTICS

In the Introduction, we presented two general types of Anxiety disorders: Primary Anxiety and Anxiety-like Disorders (ALD), both collectively referred to as Anxiety. We also developed an **analogy** for the interactions between the P&S nervous systems, which are the two branches of the ANS. We will use the analogy to help explain deeper the P&S interactions in Anxiety. Remember, the ANS is the portion of your nervous system that controls and coordinates virtually every cell in your body and certainly all of your systems. It also has the memory of your medical history. As such, we consider it to be your physiologic "fingerprint." It is, in large part, what makes you unique. Your responses and reactions go a long way to define your personality. This is part of the reason why P&S monitoring provides your doctor more information and helps to individualize your healthcare, rather than lumping you in with large groupings of "similar" patients. Individualized healthcare focuses on you individually, as opposed to 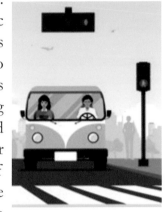 what is termed "customized" medicine which may group you with smaller groups of "similar" patients[g], but you are still grouped with many others.

The analogy associates the P&S nervous systems with the brakes and accelerator of a car that has an automatic transmission. We associated

---

g   As an example, there are approximately 90 million hypertensives in the US. Under customized medicine, four subpopulations of hypertension were defined. So, if you are a hypertensive, you are now treated like 15 million others (as opposed to 90 million); and that is supposed to make you feel better? P&S monitoring helps your doctor treat you like you, based on your own individual responses.

call many things "Anxiety," P&S monitoring helps to differentiate four (4) pathophysiologic states that present with Anxiety-like symptoms.[h] The four additional forms of Anxiety are based on P&S dysfunction that involves poor brain perfusion [42]. They include (in no particular order, but order of presentation): Sympathetic Excess, Parasympathetic Excess, Sympathetic Withdrawal, and arrhythmia.

Sympathetic Excess

Sympathetic Excess (SE, a beta-adrenergic response, see Stand response graph, right) upon standing, is associated with possible (preclinical) syncope that is the result of "adrenaline storms" that may cycle "Anxiety." When brain perfusion pressures decrease below thresholds for normal brain function, the brain signals for more blood. This signal is colloquially known as an "adrenaline storm." SE is therefore a reaction that is oftentimes not fulfilled, and syncope or pre-Syncope may result.

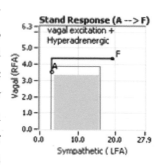

- SE and its associated syncope may be further differentiated by P&S testing and may be treated, thereby treating the Anxiety.
  - Stand SE with an abnormal stand Parasympathetic response, PE, defines Vasovagal syncope (VVS);
    - In these cases the PE is considered the primary Dyasutonomia and the SE the secondary, and it must be treated as such as to not exacerbate the SE;

---

h   Patients with anxiety-like symptoms have conditions that include the same symptoms as Anxiety, but they do not fit the definition of Primary Anxiety, or are either not fully relieved by Anxiety therapy or have documented additional dysfunction that may involve similar or the same symptoms (i.e., P&S dysfunction that causes poor brain perfusion).

the brakes with the Parasympathetics and the accelerator with the Sympathetics. As we go deeper into the different Dysautonomias that were introduced that lead to ALD, we will use the car analogy to help provide understanding. The majority of Dysautonomia patients who are diagnosed with Anxiety do not actually have a brain defect or psychological disorder. These are the ALD patients. However, that does not mean the brain is not involved. If fact, it is very much involved. It is just not defective or disordered in an anatomical or psychological sense. It is simply "sleepy" due to poor blood flow to the brain, known as poor brain perfusion.

In the Introduction we introduced two terms: Sympathetic Excess (SE) and Parasympathetic Excess (PE). These may occur together, as depicted in **Figure 3**, below, as compared with a normal response). Here we will discuss them in more detail.

Sympathetic Excess

There are resting SEs and challenge (or active) SEs. Resting SE is measured as high SB (SB = S/P at rest) and is differentiated from active SE by the label "high SB." Dynamic or active SE is measured during a Sympathetic challenge such as Valsalva or stand challenge. Primary Anxiety is typically associated with primary SE due to the mental stresses associated with the Anxiety, especially in patients that also present with high BP or hypertension. ALD is typically associated with secondary SE (secondary to PE, see below).

Both resting and active forms of SE may be secondary to other Dysautonomias that often occur upon standing or upright postural change. For example, if BP drops upon standing, SB may become high so that the increased Sympathetics may increase resting BP to compensate for the drop upon standing. For example, assume your resting (systolic) BP is normal at 110 mmHg. Assume when

- ○ Stand SE with an abnormal HR response to stand defines neurogenic syncope;
    - The cause of the abnormal HR response, typically a decrease in HR or a weak increase, needs to be investigated and treated;
- ○ Stand SE with neither of the above indicates cardiogenic syncope (a diagnosis by omission), and needs further testing to positively diagnose and determine the cardiovascular defect that is causing the (pre-)Syncope;
- ○ Combinations of the above may also exist, and is known as neurocardiogenic syncope.

Parasympathetic Excess

Parasympathetic Excess (PE, see Stand response graph, right), regardless of when it is demonstrated by P&S monitoring, may indirectly or directly compromise brain perfusion, possibly leading to "adrenaline storms" that may cycle "Anxiety." PE may be demonstrated at rest (aka, Low SB, see "Baseline" Response Graph below, left), or upon Valsalva (see Response Graph below, center)

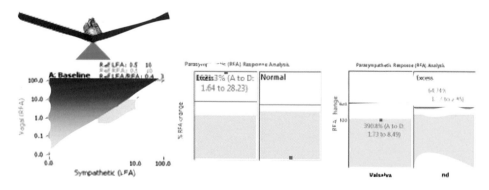

or upon stand (see Response Graphs below, right). PE may cause: resting hypotension, resting bradycardia, or insufficient rises in BP or HR with activity (challenge) causing insufficient brain perfusion. This form of ALD is also associated with Depression-like symptoms, since the brain is hypoperfused or under-perfused and

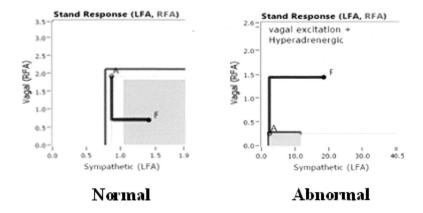

Normal   **Abnormal**

Figure 3: The normal response (left graph), as exemplified in the P&S response to standing (F) from sitting (A), is the Parasympathetics (the blue line) decrease first followed by the Sympathetics (the red line) increasing. Removing the foot from the brakes then accelerating minimizes the amount of acceleration required and potentiates the effects of acceleration. The abnormal situation of "riding the brakes" (right graph), is the Parasympathetics (the blue line) increase forcing the Sympathetics (the red line) to increase further, thereby "over-revving" the engine. This abnormal response is an example of a Vasovagal syncope response, the light-headedness often associated with Anxiety-like Disorders. Therapy should target removing the patient's foot from the brakes (Parasympathetics). This typically, organically, reduces the amount of acceleration (Sympathetics), assuming no end organ effects.

you stand, your BP should increase 10 mmHg to 120 mmHg for proper brain perfusion. However, what happens is that your BP actually decreases 10 mmHg when you stand. Eventually, what is thereby unable to function at full capacity, leading to Depression-like symptoms.

- This is an autonomic issue, further differentiated by P&S testing and may be treated, thereby treating Anxiety;
  - Treatment often includes very low-dose antidepressants, which at those dosages are low-dose anticholinergics. Normal to high doses will cause additional side-effects. While tricyclics and SNRIs are our primary recommendations, SSRIs are often preferred by most others due to their low effect on BP[i]. This is due to the fact that SSRIs have very little effect on the ANS, and therein lies the problem. In these cases, SSRIs may treat the Depression or Depression-like symptoms, but rarely do they treat the underlying Dysautonomia. More on this later in the Therapy section;
- An example of PE with (secondary SE) is presented in the Stand Response plot of Figure 3 (previous page, right), with a normal stand response to compare.

Sympathetic Withdrawal

Sympathetic Withdrawal (SW, an alpha-adrenergic response, see Stand response graph, right) upon standing (positive head-up tilt or other head-up postural change) is associated with possible (preclinical) orthostatic dysfunction. SW is documented by P&S monitoring as the red line in the Stand Response graph

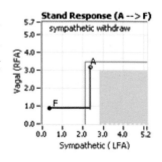

to the right, going away from the normal area of the graph (indicated in gray). SW may, directly or indirectly, compromise

---

i   At least one-third of the world's population is expected to be diagnosed with hypertension by 2023.

we see happen is that your body will reset your resting BP to 130 mmHg so that when you stand and your BP drops 10 mmHg, your BP is still at or above 120 mmHg for proper brain perfusion. Your brain remains happy. It is still getting the blood it wants. However, your heart, and therefore your cardiologist, may not be happy because you now qualify for hypertension.

Without P&S monitoring, your cardiologist will see your high BP and treat it (by treating the high SB) to return BP to normal. However, that will make your brain unhappy, and it will cause your body to defeat the anti-hypertension medication, even if your cardiologist increases your dosage or adds other medications. Your body may defeat this much medication because your body has at least seven (7) pathways to control BP and medicine is only able to block four (4), at most. So your body still has other pathways to get around the medication. Ultimately, your physician stops believing you because you insist you are taking your medication, yet your physician does not see the results that are expected. On the other hand, you may indeed avoid your medication (you may become noncompliant) because of feelings of light-headedness or dizziness, fatigue, or exercise intolerance. Either way, this may be further complicated by the fact that the anti-hypertensive therapy may make you even feel worse than before. You may become (more) exercise intolerant or return to being (more) light-headed, dizzy, brain fogged, fatigued, etc. All because the anti-hypertensive therapy actually does its job and lowers your BP again so that your brain is no longer properly perfused.

Note, the anti-hypertensives may start to compromise your heart health as well, as your heart tries to work under these multiple adverse conditions. Instead of all this as in this example, P&S

brain perfusion, through venous pooling, possibly leading to "adrenaline storms" that may cycle "Anxiety."

- SW is therefore, by definition, a vascular or blood volume issue, able to be further differentiated by P&S testing and may be treated, thereby treating "Anxiety:"
    - ○ SW with a drop in BP of 20/10 mmHg or more upon standing defines neurogenic orthostatic hypotension (NOH). SW with any other drop in BP may be considered preclinical NOH (SW is more information enabling earlier treatment);
    - ○ SW with an abnormal increase in BP in response to stand (i.e., > 30/20 mmHg BP increase) defines orthostatic hypertension, a very rare form of orthostatic dysfunction;
    - ○ SW with any other BP response to stand, including a normal BP response to stand, defines orthostatic intolerance;
    - ○ SW with an abnormal increase in HR in response to stand (i.e., > 30 bpm increase in HR or an average stand HR over 120 bpm in adults, or > 40 bpm increase in HR in children) defines postural orthostatic tachycardia syndrome (POTS);
        - ■ First-line therapy for orthostatic dysfunction includes: 1) low-dose Midodrine, titrated slowly from very low dose to enable the patient to acclimate to the new vasoconstriction, 2) proper daily hydration, and 3) high-dose antioxidant, r-ALA. For POTS, low-dose Propranolol is recommended. Propranolol has antioxidant affects, especially with high SB, and with Midodrine to blunt exaggerated HR increases with stand. Low-dose Propranolol avoids the adverse effects of reducing SE too fast.

Monitoring shows that the primary problem is not *hyper*tension (a condition documented at rest), but *hypo*tension (a condition documented during challenge[j]). Not that we do not think *hyper*tension is dangerous and needs to be treated; it is! However, in these cases, it needs to be treated in the correct manner to also treat the actual cause, the *hypo*tension. In most cases treating the *hypo*tension also (eventually) treats the *hyper*tension.

This does not preclude the primary therapy (therapy for hypotension) from also targeting the Sympathetics as secondary in order to minimize cardiovascular stress (relieve hypertension) as the two autonomic branches are normalizing. The same therapy mentioned above as not recommended as a primary therapy may be recommended (in small doses) as a secondary therapy. Secondary Sympathetic therapy may be needed to protect the systems during the healing (balancing) process. Think of it this way. Remember, the P&S nervous systems are independent systems. Therefore, if the Sympathetics are in the "habit" of over-revving the engine, this may continue for a while, even though you are removing your foot from the brakes. This will cause the car to speed up even more at first (read that HR or BP to go even higher at first). This is the result of the "bad habit" of compensating for your foot being on the brakes. Until the Sympathetics are habituated to "less brakes," therapy will be needed to prevent further harm, further over-revving; to extend this example. As we will discuss below, SE is treatable and in doing so, ALD is treated and the symptoms of Anxiety relieved.

Parasympathetic Excess

"Over-revving your engine" is exaggerating, or overstimulating your stress responses (Sympathetic responses). This may explain

---

j   Virtually all tests ordered by physicians are administered while you are resting, this is why this situation is often missed.

Arrhythmia

Arrhythmia (see the example in the Heart Rate graph, right), causes inefficient blood pumping that may compromise brain (and cardiac) perfusion, possibly leading to "adrenaline storms" that may cycle "Anxiety."

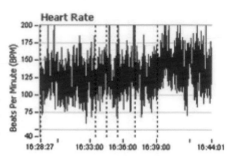

P&S monitoring elucidates the involvement of the P&S systems in the arrhythmia, helping to provide more information when developing treatment plans to relieve arrhythmia and thereby treat "Anxiety." Typically:

- High Sympathovagal Balance (SB = S/P at rest: High SB indicates a resting beta-sympathetic excess) is generally associated with Ventricular arrhythmias, but may be seen with some Atrial arrhythmias;
- Low SB (indicating a resting Parasympathetic excess) may be associated with Atrial arrhythmias;
- These are gross generalizations, for example, one study showed 80 percent of atrial fibrillation (AFib) is estimated to be autonomically mediated, and 80 percent of the autonomic subpopulation are estimated to be Parasympathetically mediated. In other words, the above assumption that AFib is Parasympathetically mediated is only (approximately) 64 percent accurate. It is Sympathetically mediated in (approximately) 16 percent of AFib patients and is cardiogenic in approximately 20 percent of AFib patients. Mainstay measures believe more AFib is Sympathetically mediated and sleep AFib is Parasympathetically mediated
    - Therapy to relieve the arrhythmia is considered first to read the rest of the nervous system and plan additional therapy as needed.

the symptoms of "Anxiety" (ALD). In Anxiety (ALD), due to PE, small worries are amplified into large worries which may become mentally crippling (commonly manifested as a panic attack).

If pain is involved, small touches become very painful responses. Instead of the Parasympathetics decreasing, as per normal, they abnormally increase (this is Parasympathetic Excess or PE), forcing the Sympathetics to increase that much further to generate the same response. This is the "amplification" process. Applying this to pain syndromes, normal stimuli (light touch and tickle) are amplified into pain responses and significant pain response may become physically crippling. This helps to explain diffuse pain syndromes such as Fibromyalgia and difficult-to manage pain syndromes such as Chronic Regional Pain Syndrome. Another example is inflammation. The Sympathetics control inflammation, so Sympathetic Excess (SE) secondary to PE may amplify the inflammatory response and may lead to excessive inflammation which may cause anaphylactic shock as an immediate response or chronic inflammation that can include many things, like arthritis, COPD, GI disorders, some autoimmune syndromes involving inflammation, or more.

Again, assuming no end organ effects (no permanent damage), typically, relieving the PE alone will eventually relieve the SE, which then reduces BP and eventually relieves the hypertension (in the Anxiety example) and other end organ symptoms. This process occurs organically over about eighteen to twenty-four months. Often, attempts to accelerate the process, by increasing dosages or adding additional pharmaceutical agents, causes more delays.

Normal

For comparison, a normal autonomic response to stand is displayed on the Stand Response graph, right. First, there is a Parasympathetic decrease (the blue line in the "Normal" graph, right) followed by a Sympathetic increase (the red line in the "Normal" graph, right). The Parasympathetics move first because they are the faster-responding branch. Further, Parasympathetic decrease potentiates and minimizes the Sympathetic response. The Sympathetic increase is an alpha-1 Sympathetic (or Adrenergic) response. The 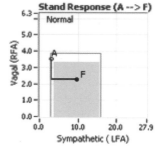 Sympathetics are the reactionary branch and the branch that is slower to respond. The Sympathetics respond based on the level of Parasympathetic activity at that moment. There is no known limit to the Parasympathetic decrease. The normal limit for the Sympathetic increase is 10 to 500 percent.

Poor Brain Perfusion

The hallmark of the P&S dysfunctions underlying ALDs is poor brain perfusion (or not enough blood flow to the brain). Actually, this includes anything above the heart and oftentimes the heart itself (see next section: High Pulse Pressure). Poor brain perfusion causes the brain or portions of the brain to function slower or "go to sleep." This makes them all primary (subclinical) Depression-like disorders. Any or all of these, together with primary Anxiety itself, may be comorbid. In general, all may be treated simultaneously, history dependent.

The lack of blood flow to the heart and structures above the heart contribute to the symptoms that accompany the P&S forms of Anxiety-like disorders. The muscles of, and between, the

Note, to use another analogy, the P&S nervous systems are like pendulums. Hitting a pendulum with a hammer to correct it only knocks it off its hinge and makes matters worse. It takes small nudges over time to correct.

To further extend the car analogy, as you are driving along, and everything is calm, what is your first reaction to a sudden, unexpected, event? . . . You hit the brakes. This is a protective response. Hitting the "brakes" or "riding the brakes" explains the symptoms of addiction, for example. Again, your body is very similar. The "brakes" (the Parasympathetics) are the protective mechanism. In addiction or compulsive behaviors, the "brakes" cause you to seek your "comfort zone" (safety), whether it be drugs, alcohol, sex, food, washing hands, or whatever is their compulsion. The Parasympathetics are strongly associated with the "Pleasure Centers" or "Comfort Centers" of the Brain stem[k] and Limbic System. Once addicted, the Parasympathetics tend to remain excessive. If the PE is not relieved during rehabilitation, then the risk of relapse remains high due to the excessive (Parasympathetic) drive to remain in your "comfort zone" stimulating their "pleasure centers."

"Riding the brakes" helps to explain other common symptoms. One is "Brain Fog" and Cognitive and Memory Difficulties: PE acts to limit the output of the heart

---

k   In the Brain stem, the Nucleus Tractus Solitarius, Nucleus Ambiguus, and Dorsal Motor Vagal Nucleus are important structures involved in efferent and afferent Vagal (Parasympathetic) activity. These nuclei are also involved in the pleasure or reward circuits of the brain, including the Nucleus Accumbens, Ventral Tegmental Area, and ultimately the Amygdala.

shoulders and of the neck are under perfused and tense up and cause pain, and may contribute to headache, including tension headache. In some cases, especially SW or PE with secondary SE, the heart is overly stressed. This may contribute to palpitations, chest pain or pressure, shortness of breath, and the feeling of having a heart attack.

Another example of the poor brain perfusion contributing to additional symptoms is that it may lead to sleep disorders, including fatigue and insomnia. Poor brain perfusion while upright throughout the day causes the brain, or portions of it, to "be asleep." This may cause fatigue compounded by the heart struggling to pump more blood to the brain. Then, when the patient lays down, gravity works, and the brain is finally properly perfused. The brain "wakes up." Now the brain "wants to play!" The patient wants to sleep. So patients lay there for hours with their brains racing, feeling more alert than during the day. This contributes to insomnia. Unfortunately, in many cases, as soon as they sit up in the morning, the thoughts they had during the night "drain away." This condition may also manifest in excessive trips to the bathroom. Again, the brain "wants to play." It "wants to go for a ride" and takes the body with it by making patients feel like they have to use the bathroom. However, on the fourth or fifth trip, as many patients report, they sit there and nothing happens. Of course not—the bladder is empty. The brain is "playing." The two questions to ask to indicate sleep difficulties due to Dysautonomia are: 1) "Does it take more than twenty minutes to fall asleep?" and 2) "Do you wake more than twice in the night, even to go to the bathroom?" If either answer is yes, then the diagnosis may be positive.

Clues to differentiating ALD from Primary Anxiety include the following and typically more than one (many times most of the following):

under stress. This results in poor brain perfusion, which results in reduced brain activity, similar to that associated with depression, but often includes hypertension. Another common symptom is fatigue. Often patients describe their fatigue as if they were "running a marathon while sitting still." Again, PE will cause this by causing normal responses to little, normal stresses to be amplified into excessive responses, including mental stresses, a minor activity, like following a recipe, becomes a major undertaking. Even sitting while engaged in a mental activity increases cardiac function, metabolism, and energy expenditure while doing little if any physical activity. The associated mental stress(es), where perception(s) is (are) reality, is (are) able to lead to these symptoms. Think of your school days where you had more than one very hard test, like final exams. After taking those hard tests, you feel very tired, like you "ran a marathon," yet you were sitting still for those four to six hours. The fatigue is due to the mental stresses you experienced consuming much of your energy[1].

A third common symptom is sleep difficulty. It is well known that chronic sleep difficulties (including both insomnia, associated with Parasympathetic Excess, and sleep apnea, associated with Sympathetic Excess) are associated with P&S dysfunction: PE may lead to daytime sleepiness, and SE may lead to nighttime sleeplessness. If you take more than twenty minutes to fall asleep, or wake more than twice a night (even to go to the bathroom), then your sleep difficulty may be caused by PE. Consider what happens when someone faints. Besides gravity working, once flat on the ground, the heart and head are at the same level. The brain is receiving

---

1   Just sitting there doing nothing, your brain consumes as much as 70 percent of the oxygen and sugars (energy) in your blood. When you perform strenuous exercise, your brain consumes up to 85 percent of your energy, controlling all of your muscles. This is the basis for fatigue from mental exertion or stress.

- Depression (often subclinical Depression) or Depression-like symptoms, especially if the patient has been medicated with antidepressants for more than three months and the therapy seems to only be managing the depression and not the P&S (i.e., if the patient misses a dose, there are significant changes in the patient's presentation);
- Light-headedness or dizziness, including fainting (Syncope) or near-fainting (feelings of fainting with the need to sit or lay down to relieve the symptoms);
- Persistent fatigue or possible chronic fatigue syndrome;
- Dehydration, especially if the patient is prescribed diuretics, or reports constantly feeling thirsty even though they report drinking plenty of water;
  - We would estimate that approximately 40 percent of our patient population is simply dehydrated, and with proper daily hydration (including fewer caffeinated, alcoholic, and sugary drinks, including drinks with artificial sugar, and including electrolytes as needed) many symptoms are relieved;
- Lower-extremity symptoms due to venous pooling or excess fluid in the tissues indicating poor circulation, including restlessness (e.g., Restless Leg Syndrome), edema, or varicose or spider veins;
- Shortness of breath with palpitations and chest tightness or chest pain without heart attack or cardiovascular disorder;
- GI upset, upper (including GERD, or persistent nausea or frequent vomiting) or lower (including frequent diarrhea, constipation, or both, or inflammation);
- Sleep difficulties;
- Frequent headache or migraine;

all the blood it wants; it's happy, you're not, but the brain is. Similarly, after being upright all day (sitting or standing) as soon as you lay down to go to sleep, your brain (which has been partially asleep all day) now has all the blood it wants; it wants to "play," you want to sleep. Patients typically report that they lay there processing their day, reviewing lists of things you could have done, should have done, or would have done, and planning for the morrow. You may also rise frequently during the night (more than twice) even to go to the bathroom, because the brain is active. It "knows" it can get you out of bed and uses that to go for a ride. Restoring proper brain perfusion (blood flow to the brain) will "wake up" the brain, process the day, and then, with the normal brain changes with evening (the serotonin-melatonin inversion), the brain will be ready for sleep at the same time you are; about two hours later.

PE with secondary SE often causes the individual to either be very calm at rest or very active when active, with very little in between. In terms of our car analogy, one is either slowly idling or else over-revving the engine, and the acceleration or stopping are abrupt, not gradual. As we will discuss below, PE is treatable and in doing so, ALD is treated and the symptoms of Anxiety relieved.

Sympathetic Withdrawal

We repeat the Stand Response graph example from above here for convenience. The graph shows the abnormality. The red (Sympathetic) portion of the response decreases (goes to the left) rather than increasing or going into the gray area (going to the right). An increase would be the normal response to cause vasoconstriction and move blood up toward the heart and the brain. The decrease, known as Sympathetic Withdrawal SW), is abnormal

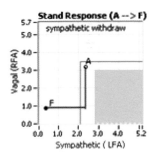

- Sensitivity to light, sound, heat, cold, touch, smells;
- Mast Cell Activation Syndrome, or allergies to foods and common items, up to and including the need for Epi-Pens;
- Generalized pain syndromes, including Small Fiber Disease;
- "Coat-hanger" pain; and
- Sexual dysfunction.

High Pulse Pressure

A possible long-term consequence of ALD due to SW may be high pulse pressures which may indicate risk of heart failure. In some cases, especially SW or PE with secondary SE, the heart is overly stressed. One stress is from the fact that the heart is not properly perfused, and therefore nourished and oxygenated. The other stress is from the brain when it issues the "adrenaline storms" causing the heart to work harder on fewer resources. Under-perfusion of the heart, whether from venous pooling due to SW or to vasodilation due to PE, results in poor cardiac return, possible poor cardiac perfusion, and lower diastolic BPs, as well as other consequences. The additional adrenaline results in the demand for higher HRs, higher cardiac output, and higher systolic BP, as well as other consequences. The two BP measures are diverging. If this divergence persists, a long-term problem may be increased, or excessive, Pulse Pressure,[m] which may lead to Heart Failure. The risk of Heart Failure increases significantly once Pulse Pressure exceeds 60 mmHg.

---

m Pulse Pressure is the difference between systolic and diastolic BP.

(and causes vasodilation which leads to the blood pooling in the feet and lower extremities (known as venous pooling). The red line, as in this graph, decreases and allows blood to move away from the heart and brain toward the feet. SW is the nerve disorder that underlies orthostatic dysfunction which is also a cause for light-headedness, fainting, brain fog, cognitive and memory difficulties, sleep difficulties, etc. There are a few forms of orthostatic dysfunction: postural orthostatic tachycardia syndrome (POTS), orthostatic hypotension (OH, including Neural OH or NOH), and orthostatic intolerance (see the physician side for further definitions). All of these disorders involve venous pooling and blood staying in the feet, leading to not enough blood in the brain (improper brain perfusion). Like with the previous two Dysautonomias (SE & PE), without proper brain perfusion, SW may also lead to the symptoms of Anxiety we discussed above. All of the conditions that are associated with SW are treatable and, in doing so, may relieve symptoms of Anxiety and ALD. As we detail in our review article [43], a cardiologist knowledgeable in P&S disorders should be part of your physician team to ensure safety and that therapy planning addresses all of your issues together.

Arrhythmia

Arrhythmia causes inefficient heart pumping and may also contribute to not enough blood in the brain (improper brain perfusion), which may contribute to the symptoms of Anxiety we discussed above (see the physician side for further discussion). As discussed on the physician side, abnormal P or S activity is often involved in arrhythmia, not just the heart. As a result, it is possible that treating P&S dysfunction in arrhythmia may also treat ALD and relieve the symptoms of Anxiety. It is important in these cases to work closely with a cardiologist knowledgeable in P&S disorders as well to ensure safety and that therapy planning addresses all of

ANXIETY INTERVENTION

An important part of any intervention with a patient with an Anxiety disorder is education. The practice guidelines recommend education of the family as well. Many people are confused and scared by the symptoms and behavior and are reassured to know they are not alone and that there are effective interventions. The patient should

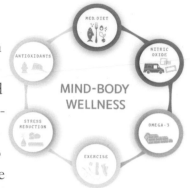

receive an appropriate medical workup, such as a physical examination, and studies (e.g., electrocardiogram, thyroid-stimulating hormone) when indicated. After ruling out a medical condition, developing a working alliance with the patient provides a basis for ongoing management and prevents further inappropriate use of the medical system.

Selective serotonin Reuptake Inhibitors (SSRIs, an antidepressant and, in low doses, an indirect anticholinergic) and Cognitive-Behavioral Therapy (CBT) are considered first-line defense for Primary Anxiety. SSRIs have been shown to be the best-tolerated medications, and response rates are significantly higher than placebo for Panic Disorder, OCD, PTSD, Social Anxiety Disorder, and GAD. SSRIs are preferred by most cardiologists due to their minimal effect on BP.[e] SSRIs and CBT also have the least potential for addiction, which is especially helpful given the prevalence of addictive behaviors noted in Anxiety patients. In all of the Anxiety disorders, SSRIs should be started at low doses and gradually titrated up to therapeutic levels to avoid an initial exacerbation of Anxiety.

However, it has been the author's experience, based on millions of P&S tests, that SSRIs have a minimal effect on the Parasympathetic your issues together. In these complex cases, addressing each symptom individually is rarely the path to wellness.

HELPFUL HINTS AND CONCEPTS

Education—An important part of any intervention with a patient with an Anxiety disorder, whether it is Primary Anxiety or P&S Anxiety, or a combination of both, is education. An understanding of why you feel anxious and what the early warning signs and symptoms are will help you to manage the Anxiety and perhaps avoid or resolve that which makes you anxious. Guidelines also strongly recommend education of the family as well. The family's education is not only to help you to recognize an anxious moment and help and support you to work yourself through that moment, but to also feel supported and useful themselves. Many people are confused and scared by the symptoms of Anxiety and behaviors that surround it (before, during, and after). Education and support from the healthcare community helps, provides comfort that something may be done, and patients as well as families are reassured to know they are not alone and that there are effective interventions.

Proper Hydration—We would estimate that upon first presentation, approximately 40 percent of our patient population is mostly just dehydrated. Remember, your body is mostly water. You live in a dry environment (the air, regardless of how humid it is). You lose water to evaporation in the dry environment. You lose water to cool yourself off. You lose water to eliminate wastes. You breathe out "a ton" of water every night while you sleep. There is more. All of this water needs to be replaced on a daily basis, and a note to the women in the audience, proper daily hydration will help to keep your hair, skin, and nails more manageable. In all of this, we mean just water. In this day and age, what most people drink is (among other things) mostly dehydrating; caffeine, sugar, fake sugar, and nervous system. This is why they have a minimal effect on BP, which is why they are preferred by most cardiologists over other anticholinergics. In cases of Anxiety not responsive to SSRIs, with P&S dysfunction or Anxiety-like symptoms, SSRIs are often discontinued and patients titrated on a very low-dose tricyclic (i.e., no more than 10 mg Nortriptyline, qd twelve hours before waking) or SNRI[n] (i.e., 20 mg Duloxetine, qd) to relieve the P&S dysfunction and treat the symptoms of ALD. Low-dose Nortriptyline may be added to SSRIs if the SSRIs are somewhat effective. Low-dose Amitriptyline may be used in place of Nortriptyline if a greater anticholinergic is needed, however, Amitriptyline has a significantly greater weight-gain side-effect.

The choice of therapies is well defined both by psychological tests and P&S monitoring, as well as other physiological tests as needed. Often however, these therapies do not completely relieve the symptoms, especially if the patient's P&S balance is not restored, both at rest and in response to challenges. The psychology therapies (including CBD) tend to be long-term, and drawn out, and the non-pharmaceutical therapies serve to create dependence between patient and therapist. As with other shortcomings of typical therapy plans for other diseases (i.e., the "statin gap"), the Mind-Body Wellness Program helps to fill the "gaps."

Unlike the commercial that says to take another medication if the primary medication is not working, stop simply treating symptoms and treat the underlying cause(s), using lower dosages and fewer medications. Lower dosages are highly recommended (assuming no end organ dysfunction) so as to not cause additional side-effects by moving the P&S nervous systems too fast or too far in the opposite direction (beyond the balance point to the opposite imbalance, such as from too little Sympathetic activity to too much).

---

n   SNRIs seem to have a greater anticholinergic effect than SSRIs.

alcohol all dehydrate. Sure, you may enjoy these sorts of drinks (we even recommend a glass of wine with dinner); however, you must drink equal amounts of water to break even, then drink 48 ounces to 64 ounces of water more to properly hydrate.

Some patients complain that they do not like the taste of water. Typically water has no, or very little, taste (assuming you have brushed your teeth). So the taste is coming from you. Consider the following.

Q: What temperature is your stomach at?
A: 98°F (approximately).
Q: What is the temperature of the water you drink?
A: Room temperature water is around 70°F, and most drink liquids at colder temperatures.
Q: What happens when you put something cold on something hot?
A: The something hot shrinks.

Even room temperature water is almost 30°F colder than your stomach. The something hot is your stomach, and it shrinks when you drink something colder. The shrinkage may cause a feeling of nausea, or fullness (satiety), or it may cause the gastric juices in your stomach to be pushed back up into your esophagus, and that is what you taste. Remember, hot coffee or hot tea are simply flavored hot water. Skip the caffeine (coffee or tea) and just drink the hot water, and your stomach will not shrink. If you wish, you may add a few drops of fresh-squeezed citrus as a flavoring, but not the store-bought additives with all of their sugars.

Exercise—is arguably the most powerful anxtioxidant available, with about twenty other benefits. By exercise we do not mean beating yourself up. That is not necessary. However, if that relieves stress, makes you happy, and is healthy for you, we are not stopping you. What we do mean is to adopt an active lifestyle, rather than sitting

Fewer medications are enabled by the fact that one medication targeted at a Dysautonomia often relieves a number of symptoms, rather than treating the multiple symptoms. For example, low-dose anticholinergic therapy may not only establish P&S balance, but it may also relieve depression, sleep difficulties, upper and lower GI upset, and more, all by balancing Parasympathetic activity, both at rest and in response to challenge.

Establish health and wellness in the nervous and cardiovascular systems. The brain and heart connection is one of the main connections between the Mind and Body. The brain and heart are connected by the P&S Nervous Systems and the vascular system. If the nervous system (including the brain) and the heart are (1) not receiving the proper amount of energy, and (2) if they are constantly fighting against the effects of stress and disease by (3) not having enough antioxidants to (4) deal with free radicals and reactive oxygen and nitrogen species so as to keep mitochondria, cell membranes, and other organelles healthy, and (5) if nitric oxide levels are low causing, among other things, (6) poor blood flow to all areas of the body and (7) not delivering these nutrients and (8) removing waste products, then Anxiety is a result. No wonder it is one of the most diagnosed diseases or disorders *in the world!*

The P&S-mediated ALDs often also involve primary or chronic diseases or disorders, including (1) most chronic diseases (the most well-known being diabetes, as well as most cardiac diseases, chronic pain, kidney disease, sleep disorders, hormone imbalances, GI disorders, respiratory dysfunction, etc.), as well as (2) significant trauma (including injury, surgery, concussion, post- and secondary concussion syndromes, and other physical and mental traumas, as in PTSD), (3) significant illnesses that lead to persistent oxidative stress (including viral and bacterial infections, and other biological at a desk all day or in front of a screen (phone, computer, television, etc.). A minimum of 150 minutes a week of moving at a rate that increases your heart rate above resting levels is what we are recommending. This may be gardening, walking, housework, actively playing with children or grandchildren, yoga, etc. Running, jogging, lifting weights, contact sports, etc., are all good as well, as long as you are fit for it.

CAUTION: As always, an exercise regimen should be started under close physician supervision. The wrong types of exercise may do more harm than good, including increasing body fat (and thereby weight), fatigue, and pain due to the fact that the body is programmed to overreact to stresses. Under these conditions, the body sees exercise as stress and works to protect itself against the stress. With certain diseases (e.g., some arrhythmias, diabetes, stroke or aneurysm risk, or heart disease), the wrong type of exercise may also lead to heart attack, stroke, or sudden death. It is best to start slow and build up and always listen to your body. Until endurance is built, recommended goals may not be reached for a while. This is not bad; keep at it until the goals are reached. The health benefits of physical activity far outweigh the risks of getting hurt.

Also, strict compliance with the recommended 150 minutes of exercise per week is not required to get beneficial effects. Smaller amounts of exercise are helpful, just not as much [44]. The twenty other benefits of exercise include: *happier moods* (brain chemicals are released that elevate mood), *reduced pain* (brain chemicals are released that relieve pain), improved *immune health* (1. simulates fever to prevent infection, and 2. is a strong antioxidant, like vitamin C but much stronger), better *sleep quality* (more restorative sleep and less daytime drowsiness, with less possibility of sleep apnea and snoring), improved *concentration & creativity* infections, even after the infection or microbe is eliminated—the result is partially damaged mitochondria with reduced energy output, but not enough to affect the resting state, only the active, or challenge, state), (4) significant exposures (environmental, chemical, temperature, radiation, etc.), and we have even found P&S dysfunctions associated with ALDs in (5) women who have had more than two pregnancies (that is any pregnancy that passed the first trimester). All of these conditions leave P&S imbalance, which perpetuates poor health and poor QoL.

SUPPLEMENTS AND LIFESTYLE MODIFICATION THERAPY: THE MIND-BODY WELLNESS PROGRAM

All six prongs of the Mind-Body Wellness Program work together to help relieve ALDs regardless of cause or form, and often relieve the burden of Primary Anxiety as well.

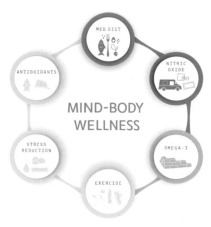

1. **Antioxidants**, vitamins, amino acids, and minerals are shown to improve, in part, depression and depression-related disorders (including Anxiety, psychosocial Stress, and obsessive-compulsive disorders) [45]. Antioxidants known to help relieve Anxiety include r-ALA[46], N-acetylcysteine (NAC) [47], Resveratrol [48], Folate° (Vitamin B$_{12}$) [49], and L-arginine [50]. Antioxidants, with these other supplements, and of course directly reducing oxidative stress [51], all help relieve oxidative stress which can be caused by, or be a cause of, ALDs, thereby helping to reduce the effects of Anxiety-like symptoms and thereby helping to maintain health and wellness.

---

o   Folate deficiency is associated with problems in cognition, mood, psychosis, and anxiety.

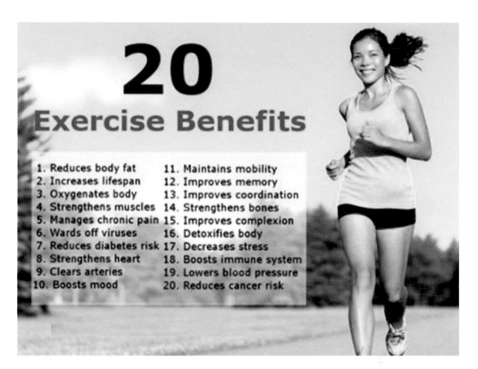

(by increasing brain perfusion), reduced *stress levels* (whole body system stress), reduced *oxidative stress* (again, **exercise** is a strong antioxidant), maintained *mental fitness* (reduces brain shrinkage), maintained *P&S balance*, improved *heart & vascular health*, improved *neuroendocrine health* (maintain healthy insulin and thyroid hormone levels, boost sex hormones and healing and repair processes, and more), aid in *weight control (loss)*, reduced Risk of *type 2 diabetes and metabolic syndrome*, reduced *cancer* risk, **detoxification** of the body, strengthening of *bones and muscles*, reduced risk of developing, and help to manage, *arthritis and other joint disorders*, maintained *mobility*, and promoted *longevity* (promotes living longer—exercise alone has never been proven to increase longevity; however, by reducing mortality risk, a patient's natural longevity is promoted or preserved).

2. **Omega-3 Fatty Acids** including Eicosapentaenoic Acid (EPA) and Docosahexaenoic Acid (DHA) [48,52,53,54,55] help relieve Anxiety-like disorders by helping to repair what chronic psychosocial and oxidative stress damages through free radical and reactive oxygen and nitrogen species [3]. Fish oil supplementation is safe and well-tolerated and, in part, has adjunctive therapeutic benefits in Anxiety and Anxiety-like syndromes without notable side effects, and with enduring benefit; including in children.

3. The unique neuromodulator **nitric oxide** influences and modulates several other conventional messengers which play an important role in Anxiety, thereby helping to reduce Anxiety [56,57].

4. **Exercise** is arguably the single most powerful antioxidant, among its many other benefits (see Patient side for list, previous page) [3].

5. **The Mediterranean Diet** provides the nutrients, including antioxidants, vitamins, minerals, amino acids, omega-3 fatty acids, nitric oxide, and their building blocks, and the energy need to power all of these activities [3]. However, diet often does not provide sufficient quantities of these elements of the Mind-Body Wellness program. Fortunately, these elements may be supplemented as needed, especially due to age or duration of disease or disorder. Part of proper dieting is to sit, relax, and enjoy a meal with friends and family with lots of laughter, and a little wine (*only one to two glasses!*). Routine and frequent episodes of this event go a long way toward reducing stress.

For exercise therapy for Dysautonomia, see Figure 4 (low and slow exercise, p. 118) and Figure 5 (supine exercises, p. 120) for the range of recommended exercises to condition your heart (not so much your skeletal muscles). Do at least one of those depicted for forty minutes a day for six months.

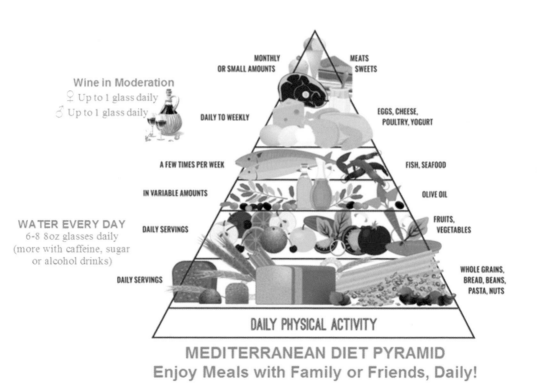

Last, but by no means less important, by reducing **psychosocial stress** itself, you relieve the many effects of Anxiety-like disorders, and perhaps Anxiety itself [3]. Some of the consequences of stress are listed in the figure below.

Our "Supplements and Lifestyle Algorithm for Dysautonomia" is presented on the patient side below, at the end of the "Helpful Hints and Concepts" section.

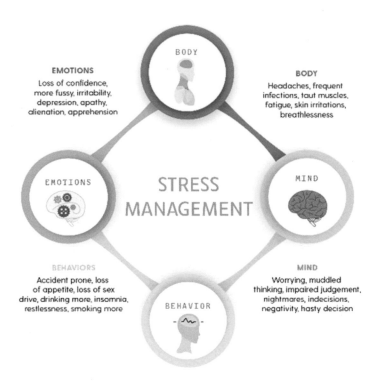

Proper diet—we recommend the Mediterranean diet, which is rich in fruits, vegetables, nuts, whole grains, fish, and seafood, and minimizes fats and red meats. It also includes a little wine! A similar diet is known as the Japomediterranean diet, since the Japanese traditionally eat a diet similar to that of the Mediterraneans. Diet not only provides the energy you need to live, but the nutrients, vitamins, minerals, proteins, amino acids, fatty acids, antioxidants, and more that you need for health and wellness. Unfortunately, as we age, our bodies make less and less of some of the essential ingredients to health and wellness. Fortunately, most of them may be supplemented. But that is all, supplemented. You still need the natural ("factory fresh"—read that farm fresh) produce and proteins so that you are also receiving all of the buffering and balancing components that make the supplements functional or optimal. For example, high doses of r-ALA, a very important and very powerful antioxidant, is best taken with a little biotin (vitamin B_8) to maintain the vitamin levels to protect from the extra acid.

Unfortunately for all too many, the American diet or Western diet is far from any diet recommended. It is a diet of convenience, a diet that is "fresh from the factory" (in this case factory does not mean farm, but a processing plant making prepackaged foods). It may be argued that the American diet is killing this country faster than anything else, especially when taken with the levels of stress under which the Western culture exists. For example, from all processed foods, one of the first things to be processed out (albeit not intentionally) is vitamin K_2. Granted, we only need small amounts of it, but it is very important. vitamin K_2 functions to redirect calcium from soft tissue to hard, like from arteries to bones. In the arteries, calcium causes coronary artery disease (CAD) and osteoporosis. This may be a reason for the high level of these two diseases in

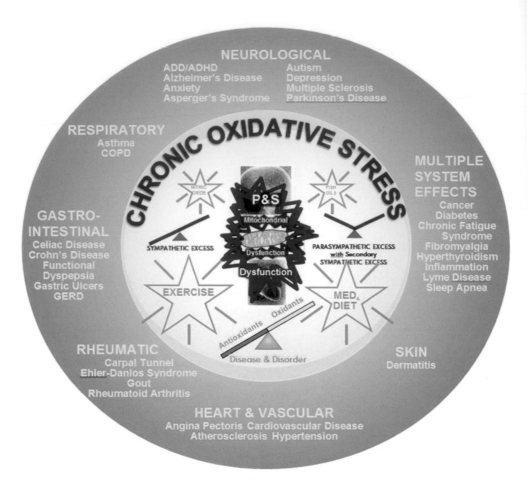

Figure: Psychosocial stress is arguably the most pervasive of all oxidative stresses, and reducing it is an antioxidant in itself. Antioxidants repair, remove, and prevent radical oxygen and nitrogen species and other free radical damage by adding electrons to all types of free radicals. The clinical manifestations of oxidative stress are numerous, some of which are listed in the outer (blue) annulus.

Western modern culture. The good news is that vitamin K_2 may be supplemented, and after about a year, much of the CAD and osteoporosis may be relieved.

Antioxidants—The effect of oxiative stress on cells and the organelles inside of cells, including mitochondria, is like is what is often seen as apples or other fruit decaying. Oxidants are breaking down the cells to help recycle nutrients. Similar events happen in your body, but normally, only with cells that are worn out. We suffer from the effects of

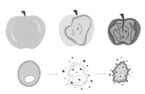

Like apples, oxidation also shrivels cells.

too much oxidation when oxidative stress persists, like after a serious illness, leaving us fatigued with no energy to do things. Yes, such patients look normal at rest, but are not able to be very active.

To combat oxidative stress, there are many antioxidants. Perhaps the most well known is vitamin C. Antioxidants serve many roles in the body, with two of the main roles being maintaining mitochondrial health to maintain optimal energy levels, and immune support in "burning the trash" that tries to infect us everyday. mitochondria produce the energy molecule that we need to live. However, mitochondria also produce "pollution" which are the oxidants (free radicals) that we take antioxidants to neutralize. The immune system actually takes this pollution (oxidants) and hands it off to invading microbes that are attempting to make you sick. In this way, the oxidants burn the trash, including viruses, bacteria, molds, mildews, allergens, and more, including the worn-out cells of our own body. Antioxidants are necessary in these situations as "fire exstinguishers," used to put out the fire once the trash is burned, before healthy tissue is burned. Many antioxidants are acids (like vitamin C, which is ascorbic

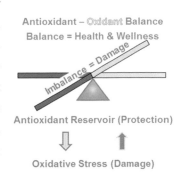

Antioxidant – Oxidant Balance

Balance = Health & Wellness

Imbalance = Damage

Antioxidant Reservoir (Protection)

Oxidative Stress (Damage)

PHARMACOLOGICAL THERAPY FOR P&S ANXIETY: HOMEOPATHIC LEVELS

The four Dysautonomias discussed above that may lead to ALDs are all treatable and in our experience, require low dose, or homeopathic dosing, of pharmacological agents to accelerate the therapy offered by the supplement and lifestyle modification recommendations of the Mind-Body Wellness Program.

Again, this book is strictly for educational purposes and is not intended to provide any medical or professional advice or diagnosis, or medical or professional opinion, or medical or professional treatment services of any kind, whether pharmaceutical, supplemental, nutraceutical, or lifetstyle, to any individual. This book shall in no way substitute or replace the patient–physician relationship or be used as a substitute for medical or professional diagnosis and treatment. Please consult a board-certified physician for medical advice or treatment and before making any decisions or changes in your healthcare treatment plan(s).

Note. One very important point is that many patients are taking central stimulants, such as Ritalin and Adderall, for treatment of so-called ADD/ADHD or other psychological or behavioral disorders. However, these patients often have Dysautonomia that impairs memory and cognitive function, often due to a lack of blood supply to their head or poor brain perfusion due to orthostatic disorders, including SW. Oftentimes, we will treat these patients with vasoactive agents (e.g., Midodrine, Pyridostigmine, or Droxidopa) first to see if their cognition improves and brain fog lessens before even considering them for treatment with central stimulants by psychiatry. In the United States, Methylphenidate is classified as Schedule II controlled substance. It is recognized to have medical value but presents a high potential for abuse.

Acid, and r-ALA). So care must be taken not to take too much. Yet, still to protect mitochondria and to maintain immune health, a proper antioxidant balance that leaves a little bit of oxidant in the body is healthful, however, the body also needs a ready reserve of antioxidants "banked" and ready to go at a moment's notice when needed.

Nitric Oxide—Nitric Oxide also offers many benefits to the body. It may act as an antioxidant, a anti-inflammatory, an antisclerotic (preventing and reducing cholesterol built up in the arteries), and an anti-hypertensive by dilating blood vessels. It maintains endothelial health to enable blood to flow smoothly and help things pass into and out from cells as is normal. It is a universal messenger, a Parasympathetic nerve transmitter, and more [3].

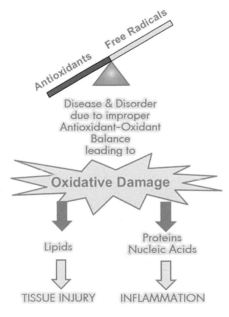

There are two main pathways by which the body produces nitric oxide. One is through the amino acid pathway with L-arginine, of which L-carnitine and C-citrulline may be used to make L-arginine. Further, L-arginine does not pass through the stomach well, but the other two amino acids do, and lastly, L-arginine is rate limited. Once the body has what it needs, it stops producing L-arginine. The other pathway is through the mouth and stomach. The friendly bacteria that live there are happy to provide us with as much nitric oxide as we are able to feed them oral nitrates. Currently, the most common source of nitrates is beet root powder extract.

Sympathetic Withdrawal—SW & PE are the two most prevalent Dysautonomias in P&S Anxiety. As mentioned before, SW is associated with venous pooling, leading to poor venous return to the heart and thereby poor brain perfusion. It is also the disorder that is associated with orthostatic dysfunction, including OI, OH, & POTS. The primary treatment for SW is r-ALA with proper daily hydration.

Midodrine, First-Line Pharmaceutical Treatment

Primary treatment recommended for SW is 2.5 mg, tid, Midodrine, titrated slowly to minimize the new vasoconstriction side-effects: starting with 1.25 mg every other morning for two weeks, then 1.25mg every morning for two weeks, then 2.5 mg every morning for two weeks, then 2.5 mg every morning and noon and finally 2.5 mg tid.

Midodrine, Side Effects

The most frequent side-effects of Midodrine are piloerection ("goose bumps" on the skin), chills, scalp pruritus ("itchy" or "crawly" scalp), numbness and tingling (paresthesias) on the face or throughout the body, and urinary retention or, at times, urethra discomfort, especially in males with benign prostatic hypertrophy. Please note that these symptoms are indications that the medicine is working. We understand that these symptoms may be overwhelming. That is why we highly recommend that the prescribed dosage be titrated very slowly, perhaps over as much as three months. We found this to be especially necessary in cases where patients have been previously prescribed high doses of Midodrine (10mg or more tid).

Many patients are frightened by the initial side-effects of Midodrine. Patients may need multiple reassurances that these are really not side-effects, but may be an indication that the vasoconstriction is actually working. We emphasize that we are encouraged to see these

Omega-3 Fatty Acids—Also perform multiple functions in the body. They are the primary building blocks for cell walls, helping to keep cell walls flexible and thereby facilitate transport into and out of cells. This activity in Endothelial cells helps to promote the activty of nitric oxide, as summarized above. This activity in the myelin sheaths that surround nerve cells to help them funciton more efficiently helps to maintain healthy nerve cells. This helps the body's cognitive function stay sharper, stabilize mood, and maintain muscle coordination. Omega-3 fatty acids are anti-sclerotic in that they reduce and prevent the buildup of cholesterol plaque on the walls of arteries, thereby helping to reduce or prevent atherosclerosis. This enhances circulation. They are anti-inflammatory, helping to reduce S-activity.

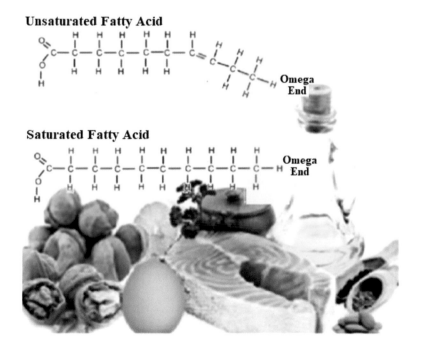

reported symptoms, which reassures the patient has been compliant, it is being absorbed, and it is working to restore vasoconstriction. For those without SW, vasoconstriction is common, frequent, and largely ignored; like the shirt on your back. Until it was just mentioned, you are mostly unaware of your shirt. This is the new normal we are promoting with vasoconstriction. You and your patients need to become used to it.

Very little Midodrine crosses the Blood-Brain Barrier. However, occasionally, headaches have been reported, especially in the beginning, due to some of its vasoconstrictor effects. This may include additional head pressure due to more blood flow to the head and brain.

Midodrine, Adjunctive Therapy

Volume expanders may be needed to maintain proper hydration. If the patient reports drinking 48 to 64 ounces of water a day, but spilling it almost immediately, then they may need assistance keeping the fluid in their vessels. Desmopressin may be recommended at 0.1 mg or 0.2 mg once a week to build volume. For females, an additional dose during menstruation, as needed, is often helpful. Fludrocortisone is the other volume expander we have used. There may be problems with Fludrocortisone [58], including possible long-term use causing fibrosis. Therefore, take care in prescribing Fludrocortisone, and only prescribe it if further therapy is needed, adjunctive to Midodrine. Fludrocortisone potentiates the effects of Midodrine, and vice versa, enabling lower dosages of both when used together, thereby limiting the side-effects of both agents. Midodrine may lower HR, especially with alpha-Adrenergic blocking agents or beta-blockers. In these cases, HR should be monitored carefully. Oftentimes, this is beneficial and welcomed, as many patients with OI disorders have a form of POTS with high HRs (about ⅓ in our experience). With Midodrine, another warning for patients is to avoid over-the-counter drugs, such as pseudoephedrine or other

Two of the main types of omega-3 fatty acids are Docosahexaenoic Acid (DHA), and Eicosapentaenoic Acid (EPA). These two chemicals go into the cell membranes of the body and help the membranes and all the cells work better. In the cardiovascular system, high-dose omega-3s (1.8g or more), primarily EPA, have been shown to reduce cardiovascular events and close the "statin gap," reducing the cholesterol left behind by statins. With their anti-inflammatory properties, omega-3 fatty acids may help with Asthma, ADHD, Cognitive difficulties, improve some cancer prognoses (e.g., colorectal, non–small cell lung, pancreatic, and breast), help with Crohn's Disease and Inflammatory Bowel Diseases, help reduce Periodontitis and Gingivitis, Depression, and Psoriasis, improve management of Lupus and Rheumatoid Arthritis.

Stress Reduction—In addition to reducing oxidative stress (see antioxidants above), which is stress at the cellular level, Stress needs to be reduced at the system and whole-body level. Whole-body level stress reduction is the focus here. Stress reduction comes in many forms: exercise, prayer and meditation, play, time with friends or family, and more. In fact, anything that reduces Sympathetic activity and promotes Parasympathetic activity helps to reduce stress.

Deep Breathing is a technique by which an individual relaxes while breathing at six breaths per minute or inhales very slowly (without totally filling your lungs) for five seconds and then exhales very slowly for five seconds, and repeats this five more times. On average, this is the most powerful stimulus for the Parastmpathetic nervous system. It is part of the P&S test and may be used in most situations. For example, with Anxiety patients, being coached through a minute of Deep Breathing often helps you recover from a Panic Attack more quickly.

Breathing techniques are a hallmark of many other stress-reduction alpha-Adrenergic agonists. The optimal morning dose of Midodrine is 5 to 10 minutes before rising, right at the bedside to counter early morning (severe) symptoms. The final dose should be taken three (3) to four (4) hours before lying down, including in bed. We generally prescribe for 8am, 12pm, and 4pm. This may vary depending time of waking.

Mestinon, Second Line Pharmaceutical Treatment

In case patients are unresponsive or still overwhelmed by Midodrine, the second-line therapy is low-dose Mestinon, 30 mg, tid, titrated to 60mg if needed. Take care if the patient reports constipation as that is one of the side-effects of Mestinon. While Mestinon is considered to be vasoactive, it does not cause the vasoconstriction side-effects of Midodrine, and in that regard is more well tolerated. However, Mestinon has many other side-effects, making it the second-line therapy.

Maintenance Dosing

Midodrine should only be considered when non-pharmacologic strategies (e.g., high-dose r-ALA [11]) with or without volume expanding drugs have failed to alleviate symptoms. Ultimately, the recommended plan is to discontinue the pharmaceuticals and reduce the r-ALA to a maintenance dose of 200 mg, tid, with fluids. Therapy is designed to retrain the alpha-adrenergic system to respond properly, and once retrained, assuming no end organ effects, may carry forward therapy-free. An expectation of this is that, although a vasopressor, once Midodrine (or any other SW therapy) is successful, the lower vasculature should be reintegrated with the heart, reducing cardiac workload. The decreased cardiac workload will be measured as a decrease in, and perhaps normalization of, resting BP (remember, it may have been high to compensate for the orthostatic drop upon standing). SW is often, initially, masked by PE. If standing BP is abnormal or standing Tachycardia techniques, including biofeedback or neurofeedback techniques[p] (see "neurofeedback" below, on the physician side), cognitive behavioral therapy, yoga, tai chi, and the like. Other stress-reduction techniques include acupuncture and massage.

Note, with the use of Anticholinergics in P&S Anxiety, the use of Benzodiazepine and other tranquilizers are strongly discouraged.

These last six recommendations are of course from the Mind-Body Wellness Program and are all considered equally important. No one should be excluded. They all work together to form a whole that is greater than the sum of their parts. Add to these six the education, proper daily hydration, and address any sleep difficulties (see next subsection below), and you have a powerful arsenal to combat Anxiety.

Sleep difficulties—as discussed above, when you have been upright all day and your brain is under-perfused due to the autonomic symptoms of P&S Anxiety, then you lay down to go to sleep, it is like fainting. Now your brain has all of the blood it wants and is ready to "play." Mild to moderate exercise within about two hours before bedtime will help through two mechanisms. One, if you have any edema or venous pooling, it will move that excess fluid out of your legs and reduce the occurrence of Restless Leg Syndrome that may inhibit restorative sleep. Two, exercise will raise your body temperature (like simulating a fever). The return to normal body temperature will relax you and help you to fall asleep. Improved and restorative sleep goes a long way toward helping with Anxiety (and Depression).

---

p Biofeedback uses HR or HR variability (HRV), for example, as a means of training the nervous system to relax. Neurofeedback uses EEG waves (from your brain) as a means of training the nervous system to relax. Neurofeedback requires trained healthcare professionals to train the patient, and interpret and assess the outcomes. Biofeedback does not.

is documented, then we suspect SW and prescribe it with therapy for PE.

Midodrine is a first-line drug for the treatment of OH. We use it also as a first-line drug for treatment of POTS, OI syndromes in general, and VVS. Midodrine should be prescribed and titrated under the auspices of an experienced specialist who has used this in the past for Autonomic Dysfunction syndromes.

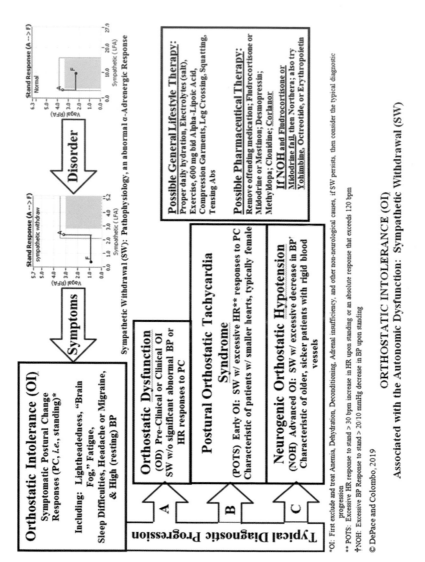

With or without exercise, assuming a 15° *Head Down Posture*[q] for 20 minutes, two hours before bedtime will also help you to sleep. This will help to move blood (and any extra fluid) from your feet to your heart to be recirculated and up to the brain to "wake up" the brain. Doing this two hours before sleep gives your brain time to process your day, go through the normal-day-to-night conversion (the serotonin-melatonin inversion[r]), and you fall asleep naturally. This may take up to a couple of weeks, depending on how long you have had the problem, but you should begin to fall asleep faster (in under 20 minutes) and stay asleep more soundly (waking no more than twice a night even to go to the bathroom).

To assume a head-down posture, take, for example, a three-cushion couch. Remove an end cushion and stack it on top of the other end cushion (see below). Lying on your back, put your feet on the stack, your bottom on the middle cushion, and your head in the hole left by the cushion you removed (perhaps with a little pillow to support your neck) and lay there for twenty

15° Head-Down Posture

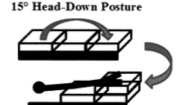

---

q   Only 15° is recommended, this is sufficient to move blood, but not too much to stretch joints, especially for EDS, Hypermobility, or Arthritis patients.

r   In the brain, serotonin puts you to sleep and melatonin wakes you up. Serotonin is why Grandma's or Great-Grandma's recommendation of warm milk works. There is serotonin in milk that is liberated by warming it. This serotonin crosses into the brain (across the blood-brain barrier) and helps to raise serotonin levels a little, just higher than the melatonin levels (this is the inversion) to put you to sleep. Melatonin does not cross the blood brain barrier, and of course is activated by sun light to wake you up (and give you a tan from the melatonin in your skin). When you take extra melatonin for something like jet lag, the brain senses more melatonin outside the brain, thinks enough has been made, and reduces melatonin production inside the brain; just enough to be a little lower than the serotonin levels and you fall asleep (defeating jet lag, in the example).

Symptoms of PE

PE is associated with some or all of the following: difficult-to-control BP, blood glucose, hormone level, or weight, difficult-to-describe pain syndromes (including CRPS), unexplained arrhythmia (palpitations) or seizure, temperature dysregulation (both response to heat or cold and sweat responses), and symptoms of depression or anxiety, ADD/ADHD, fatigue, exercise intolerance, sex dysfunction, sleep or GI disturbance, light-headedness, cognitive dysfunction or "brain fog," or frequent headache or migraine. Given that the Parasympathetics are the protective branch of the ANS, PE represents a state where the Parasympathetics regard everything as a stress and is overreacting to protect the body. This is another reason for therapy being low dose and slow.

Parasympathetic Excess—PE is the other most common Dysautonomia associated with P&S Anxiety. To review, PE is an abnormal Parasympathetic response to a Sympathetic or stress challenge. PE causes a secondary SE. PE is always the primary Dysautonomia and must be treated as such, with SE as the secondary. Again, as above, PE often masks SW, and treating PE unmasks SW and exacerbates symptoms, including light-headedness. The main clue to whether SW is masked is an abnormal BP response to stand (including a slight decrease in BP upon standing, when a 10 percent increase is expected), or an excessive HR response to stand. So we either (1) prepare to prescribe Midodrine for SW when it becomes unmasked, especially if the patient is concerned about too much medication or has a history of medication sensitivity, or (2) because SW is usually unmasked prior to a follow-up visit, we provide the patient with a prescription for Midodrine at the first visit. Midodrine is still the first-line pharmacetucal treatment, following ALA and daily hydration.

minutes (reading or watching television, but not sleeping). Again, this will help to move blood from your feet to your head and wake up the brain so you may sleep more soundly and have a better chance at restorative sleep to help relieve Anxiety (and Depression).

Caution: If at any time during this twenty minutes you feel extra head pressure or headache, stop immediately. Head pressure is not a good thing. This only means that your brain is not used to the extra blood and you may need a few times to work up to twenty minutes. This is okay. Take your time. Like everything else with P&S therapy, small changes over time is the plan so as to not cause any other problems.

Note: Do not exceed twenty minutes in the head-down posture, or else your lazy P&S nerves will think that gravity is doing the work for them, and they will remain lazy. Yes, you want to be head up through the night to make those lazy nerves work a little all night long, as part of the "retraining program." So, head up to sleep and head down to induce sleep. Also, twenty minutes (head-down posture) to prevent laziness, and forty minutes (for exercise) to push through laziness (the lethargy or resistance the body makes that you must *gently* push through to retrain the nervous system). Helping to pattern sleep is usually the first sign that the Nortriptyline therapy is working to help relieve your P&S Anxiety. We look for this, and this is why we prescribe the dosing of it for twelve hours before waking.

The Supplement and Lifestyle Therapy Algorithm for Dysautonomia figure below helps to summarize our Helpful Hints and Concepts that we have developed to help our patients reestablish a more normal quality of life and productive lifestyle.

Nortriptyline, First-Line Pharmaceutical Therapy

Therapy specific to PE is, of course, Anticholinergic therapy. Anticholinergic therapy is very low-dose antidepressant therapy. The first-line Anticholinergic therapy that we recommend is 10.0 mg, Nortriptyline, qd, 12 hrs before waking. If the patient is a blue-collar worker or other whose job may be jeopardized by a tricyclic prescription or is intolerant of or unresponse to Nortriptyline, we recommend 20 mg, qd, Duloxetine. Very rarely do we ever exceed these dosages to prevent therapy-induced symptoms, and again, when necessary, we titrate slowly. The twelve hours before waking is in response to our observations that patients reported fatigue if waking (to an alarm clock, for example) before the twelve-hour period had passed from time of dosing. However, once the twelve hours ended, patients reported being alert. We moved dosing back from bedtime to the twelve hours and patients reported refreshing sleep and no need for alarms. While anticholinergic therapy takes some months to effect PE, one of the first results is that these two agents will begin to pattern sleep. With refreshing sleep in about two weeks, patients report beginning to feel better and are encouraged.

We prefer Nortriptyline in most cases because it has the least weight-gain effect and, at the low doses, it has little effect on BP. However, in cases where the patient seems to be underweight, we will consider 10.0 mg, Amitriptyline, qd, twelve hours before waking. Amitriptyline is a more potent anticholinergic, and has a greater weight-gain effect. Care must be taken in cases of hypertension or Cardiovascular Disease (CVD) and when beta-blockers are involved. This does not include POTS patients (see below). If the patient may need or is prescribed a beta-blocker, we recommend prescribing or switching to dose-equivalent or lower Carvedilol. Carvedilol is a double cocktail, including both an alpha- and a beta-agent. This combination has been found to have antioxidant properties and helps to relieve PE as well as SE.

SUPPLEMENT AND LIFESTYLE THERAPY ALGORITHM FOR DYSAUTONOMIA

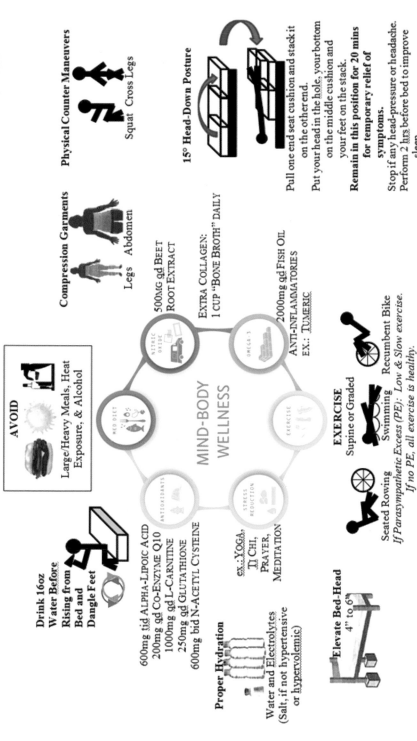

Physical Counter Maneuvers

Squat   Cross Legs

15° Head-Down Posture

Pull one end seat cushion and stack it on the other end.
Put your head in the hole, your bottom on the middle cushion and your feet on the stack.
Remain in this position for 20 mins for temporary relief of symptoms.
Stop if any head-pressure or headache.
Perform 2 hrs before bed to improve sleep

DO NOT PERFORM WITHIN 2 HRS TO 4 HRS OF TAKING MIDODRINE, DEPENDING ON DOSAGE

Compression Garments

Legs   Abdomen

AVOID
Large/Heavy Meals, Heat Exposure, & Alcohol

500MG qd BEET ROOT EXTRACT

EXTRA COLLAGEN: 1 CUP "BONE BROTH" DAILY

2000mg qd FISH OIL
ANTI-INFLAMMATORIES
EX.: TUMERIC

NITRIC OXIDE

OMEGA-3

MED DIET

MIND-BODY WELLNESS

EXERCISE

ANTIOXIDANTS

STRESS REDUCTION

EXERCISE
Supine or Graded

Recumbent Bike

Swimming

Seated Rowing

*If Parasympathetic Excess (PE): Low & Slow exercise.
If no PE, all exercise is healthy.*

Drink 16oz Water Before Rising from Bed and Dangle Feet

600mg tid ALPHA-LIPOIC ACID
200mg qd CO-ENZYME Q10
1000mg qd L-CARNITINE
250mg qd GLUTATHIONE
600mg bid N-ACETYL CYSTEINE

ex.: YOGA,
TI CHI,
PRAYER,
MEDITATION

Proper Hydration

Water and Electrolytes (Salt, if not hypertensive or hypervolemic)

Elevate Bed-Head
4" to 6"

Proper Exercise and Hydration are most important for long-term relief

We understand that this is a lot, but there is a lot going on with you, so let's get started!

© DePace and Colombo, 2019

113

Low and Slow Exercise, An Adjunctive or Alternate Therapy

In cases where Anticholinergics are not tolerated or not wanted, or as an adjunct to Anticholinergics, we recommend exercise. However, like any other Autonomic therapy, in these cases exercise must also be low dose and slowly titrated. The primary goal is to recondition the heart. The skeletal muscles may be well conditioned, but the heart may not be, especially if the patient would exercise (usually) heavily and often. They were doing so because they felt better. They felt better because their skeletal muscles were helping their heart to pump and circulate blood. Often the problem is that after their exercise, they would "crash." Their hearts could not keep up, and once they stopped the exercise period, their brain (and possibly their heart) would become under-perfused. This is manifested on occasion (especially in women) when they report feeling great in the gym, but nearly fainting in the locker room afterward, or in the shower, where they sometimes actually faint.

Again, this exercise is low and slow from a skeletal muscle perspective and intensive from a cardiac perspective. Because with PE, moderate to strenuous exercise has become a stress for the patient and will only exacerbate PE. Therefore, for six months, only zero-impact, pure cardiac workouts (e.g., long, easy walks at about two miles per hour, or very easy bike rides, or walking in a pool with the water level above the belly button) to avoid any tissue breakdown or stress that will stimulate Parasympathetic activity, and to avoid (at first) any significant

REASONS WHY YOU MAY HAVE BEEN MISDIAGNOSED OR POORLY MANAGED

TWO IMPORTANT FACTS

First, please understand two important facts. Fact number one: doctors are not taught about the P&S nervous systems from a clinical point of view. Until P&S monitoring was used through the late 2000s and into the 2010s, there simply was no data upon which to teach them anything. The first chapter on anything to do with the P&S nervous systems did not appear in any medical school primers until the late 2000s, and that only focused on orthostatic hypotension (OH), and that only from what was known from tilt-table testing. Unfortunately, tilt-table testing is a measure of only total autonomic activity and forces assumption and approximation to theorize P&S. The results were all about the hypotension, the change in BP. Unfortunately, a lot was missed, including how to produce highly reliable and repeatable clincial outcomes in a standard street clinic (as opposed to a research hospital). However, it was better than nothing. Granted, OH is considered the most debilitating of the Dysautonomias [12,13], but it is only one of many. The first book on clinical P&S dysfunction was not published until 2014. Without the clinical outcomes data, there was nothing to teach.

increases in HR or BP that may be interpreted by the nervous system as a stress and exacerbate PE. Although very easy elliptical machine workouts, or swimming, etc., are also zero-impact, these modalities tend to elevate HR & BP too fast, causing additional stress in these patients. The standard is walking at 2 mph for forty contiguous minutes. If you wish to swim, do not use arms and legs at the same time. When you use your legs (with a kickboard), kick as if walking at 2 mph. When you use your arms, swim very slowly, again low and slow exercise. Involving too many muscles at the same time causes HR to rise too fast, and that is the stress indicator. Biking is acceptable if you pedal like walking at 2 mph. The goal is to only stimulate, gently, Sympathetic activity and retrain the autonomic nervous system to react normally to stresses. This exercise must be for forty minutes per day (you may need to work up to this) every day for six months. Remember, a habit has been formed which must now be broken and a new habit formed to replace it. Target HR or BP is not the goal. For example, after forty minutes of walking, the patient should be able to carry on a normal conversation without being winded. They will still have increased HR and BP and sweated, but perhaps not within the first fifteen to twenty minutes. Skipping a week starts the six months over again. After the six months and a normalization of Parasympathetic activity, activities that might damage tissue (more strenuous exercises) may be returned. In this way, the Parasympathetics are (re)trained to not overreact to stressful stimuli, making for a more normal autonomic response.

Fact number two, you cannot give a clinical doctor a problem without a solution—a recognized, reliable, repeatable, positive clinical outcome. They do not have time for research. The data were not collected and published until 2014. (It took thirty years to compile and document.) Further, there are only two medications that are FDA approved for autonomic therapy (let alone P&S therapy), Midodrine and Droxidopa, and the second was not approved until 2014; and again, both drugs are only approved for OH or, in the case of Droxidopa, NOH, but still OH or a more limited version of it. Both are narrow applications. As a result, most therapies for Dysautonomia are off-label, making it even more difficult for the nonspecialist. For this reason, and the fact that a primary, first-line medication for many Dysautonomias is Midodrine, treatment of Dysautonomia should be prescribed and titrated under the auspices of an experienced specialist who has successfully relieved Autonomic Dysfunction syndromes.

THE PROBLEM IS NOT ONLY THAT IT IS NOT IN YOUR MIND BUT IT IS ALSO NOT WHILE YOU ARE AT REST

The result of the above and more, as we'll discuss, leads to frequent misdiagnoses or incomplete diagnoses. A primary reason for misdiagnoses is the office visit assessment. The majority of the time, physicians assess patients while they are sitting or laying down, while they are resting. Therefore, their treatment is to relieve your condition while you are resting.

LOW AND SLOW EXERCISE
Supine or Graded

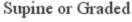
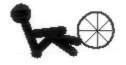

Seated Rowing   Swimming   Recumbent Bike
If Parasympathetic Excess (PE): Low & Slow exercise.
If no PE, all exercise is healthy.
Figure 4

In cases where the patient cannot rise from the bed, exercise is still strongly recommended. However, in these cases, supine exercise is the recommendation. Rolling to the floor from the bed and with the back flat on the floor, their bottom against the bed and their knees on top of the bed, have the patient move their lower legs as if they are walking at 2 mph. In this position, blood will flow from the feet and legs to the heart and then to the brain. The patient will tolerate the exercise and the heart will be engaged in conditioning. Patients may still need to work up to forty minutes. Counsel the patients to stop immediately for that day if they feel any head pressure or additional headache due to the increased blood flow to the brain for which they are not yet acclimated. As cardiac conditioning improves, the patient may lift their head off the floor for as long as possible or up to forty minutes. The third step is to do inverted bicycle exercises for up to forty minutes. At this stage, the entire forty minutes may be filled with any combination of these supine exercises

Most Dysautonomias do not present symptoms (only) at rest. They are mostly dynamic dysfunctions. By the time we tend to see patients, they have been to more than a dozen and a half physicians (including psychiatrists) for over a decade or more, searching for answers to their problems, and all others are telling them that they are normal and, by that time, that the problem is in their head. So we show them on their P&S test report that the other physicians are correct. They are normal at rest. They better be—they have had a large number of doctors working very hard to get you normal . . . at rest.

Therein lies the problem. The Dysautonomia manifests while active. To extend the car analogy (perhaps too far, sorry): many Dyasutonomias are like having a full fuel tank, but a clogged fuel line. So while idling (at rest), everything works well, but step on the gas to be active, and the engine "mushes-out." Acceleration is slow, and activity is sluggish, because even with plenty of fuel, none is making it to the engine. So you stomp on the gas harder and finally go, but are over-revving the engine. Thus the two states: resting or over-revving, even though you are going nowhere fast. P&S monitoring documents the resting state, proving what you knew all along—it is not in your head, it is in your body—and now we are looking in the right directions. This is the reason for the longer test and a test with activities. The Deep Breathing challenge simulates times when you are preparing for sleep (sleep is a very dynamic and complicated state) or after a large meal or resting. The Valsalva challenge simulates times of exercise or stress or activity. The stand challenge (or upright posture challenge if you are wheel chair bound) not only elucidates causes of light-headedness (or dizziness), but also documents whether the two P&S branches are coordinating correctly. If they cannot coordinate for something as common as sitting up or standing, they are certainly

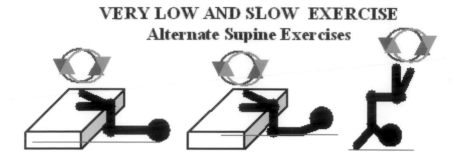

VERY LOW AND SLOW EXERCISE
Alternate Supine Exercises

Figure 5

Sympathetic Excess—SE, if comorbid with PE, is always secondary to PE and must be treated as such or else the patient will become noncompliant due to increasing symptoms, or the patient's body will defeat the sympatholytic because there are more Sympathetic pathways than medicine is able to block. Therefore, SE therapy is case specific, and unless there is an immediate threat from prolonged SE, SE may not need to be treated. This assumes there is time and safety to wait for PE relief and thereby the eventual, organic relief of SE. While SE therapy is case specific, here are some generalities to consider when working to relieve the Anxiety symptoms.

If the patient is diagnosed with POTS, and frequent tachycardia is documented and confirmed (e.g., by Holter monitor), then we recommend low-dose Propranolol (10 mg to 20 mg, bid) or some other beta-blocker with little to no effect on BP, as adjunctive to ALA and possibly Midodrine as described above.

If the patient is diagnosed with high SB, then SE therapy is based on history and whether HR or BP is high, unless they are also diagnosed with PE. If the latter, then low-dose Carvedilol is recommended as adjunctive, titrated as needed.

not coordinating properly when controlling the heart, brain, or other organs and systems of the body. These are misdiagnoses, because most doctors are not trained to look in the right places.

Case Complexity

Another reason for misdiagnoses is that the vast majority of Dysautonomia patients are complex cases. Until medicine learns the earlier warning signs of P&S dysfunction, prior to Dysautonomia (or permits periodic, preventative P&S testing), by the time most Dysautonomia patients are seen, they have more than one autonomic dysfunction and their cases are already complicated. The longer the time before recognition or diagnosis, the more Dysautonomias they tend to have. As one wise medical school professor was fond of saying: "Your patient, in the processes of their disorder or disease, had to go up and over a mountain to get to you; the best you will do is to help them back up and over the same mountain. Unfortunately, there are no tunnels to be dug."

Furthermore, physicians are trained or directed today to simply write prescriptions for symptoms: one symptom, one medication. There is rarely time or interest to listen and consider to the complaint in light of the history and deduce only one or two underlying causes. Unfortunately, with multiple medications, additional symptoms are created. The typical training is Symptom A → Drug B, Symptom C → Drug D. By the time we get to Symptom E, the training is a knee-jerk reaction: → Drug F. There is no longer a pause to consider if drugs B or D are involved in symptom E; and this only gets worse with more drugs. Another way to think of this is to consider the old nursery rhyme: "I know an old lady who swallowed a fly. She swallowed a spider to catch the fly, then a cat, then a dog, then . . ." Simply bigger and bigger things to catch the previous thing she swallowed.

Arrhythmia—high quality arrhythmia artificially inflates all HRV (total autonomic) measures, and is contraindicated. This is not the case for P&S monitoring. While high-quality arrhythmia does change how P&S reports are read, they still do contain P&S information. If SB is high, then the arrhythmia has a Sympathetic component. If SB is low, then the arrhythmia has a Parasympathetic component. Treat the cause of the arrhythmia, including any P&S dysfunction, clear the arrhythmia, if possible, and read the rest of the nervous system.

As mentioned, arrhythmia may be cardiogenic or neurogenic (or both). If neurogenic, then the arrhythmia may be Parasympathetic or Sympathetic. In both cases, treating the underlying autonomic cause often relieves the arrhythmia, and thereby relieves the Anxiety symptoms.

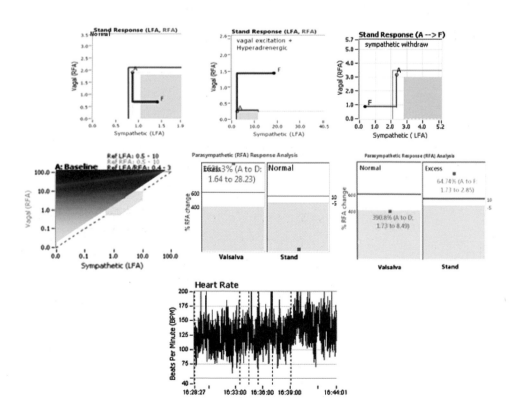

You would think that before swallowing the blue whale to catch the elephant, someone might consider going in and getting that darn fly! True, we exaggerate, but when we see patients on fifteen to seventeen medications a week and they look like lumps in a chair, consigned to "being old," we have to wonder what we are doing to our patients.

External Non-Physician Factors Restricting Physicians' Time and Options

The lack of time taken by physicians to assess patients and to think "outside the box" is also a result of medicine being commandeered by lawyers and insurance companies. Lawyers tend to target physicians who do not follow "accepted" or "standard" protocols, so many Physicains are leery about thinking outside the box. More and more, insurance companies are dictating what doctors can and cannot do by arbitrating what they will and will not reimburse. As a result, many physicians are forced to donate a quarter to a third of their practice to be able to uphold their Hippocratic Oath and treat the patient in front of them, or simply turn patients away if they cannot pay in a private-pay model. The pharmaceutical companies are also involved, in that they govern most of what is taught in medical school. Remember, they are not in business to make you well or even healthy; they are in business to sell drugs. Lastly, you, the patient, are also involved. Granted, research is good and helps you to work better with your doctor and understand your disorder better, but a (relatively) brief education from the internet (which is already limited to what is accepted) does not make you an expert. Further, many of you are convinced that you need a particular agent, and if you are not prescribed it, you will find a physician who will prescribe it. All in all, these issues lead to the physician losing in one way or another and often having to go against training to survive and treat those who will comply.

ANXIETY RISKS: DEPRESSION AND SUICIDE

The hallmark of P&S Anxiety is PE with SE or SW. PE & SW lead to subclinical depression due to poor brain perfusion and SE is the result of "adrenaline storms" that lead to Anxiety. Primary Anxiety is also associated with SE. Either way, SE is dangerous and increases both morbidity and mortality risk, including major adverse cardiovascaulr events (MACE) risk and risk of sudden cardiac death. For example, SE results in platelet activation, hemodynamic stress, oxidation of LDL, chronic inflammation, high BP, ventricular arrhythmias, and more. SE is a direct result of persistent or chronic stress of any sort, mental or physical.

According to a recent study (circa. 2018 [59]), more than one-third of American adults may be using prescription medications that can potentially cause depression or increase the risk of suicide. These prescription medications include: hormonal birth control pills, heart and BP medications, proton pump inhibitors, antacids, and painkillers. There are over two hundred commonly used prescription drugs that have depression or suicide listed as a potential side-effect. Because of their wide use, doctors are often unaware of any increased risk of depression or suicide, even though they are known side-effects. Approximately 15 percent of adults who used three or more of these medications at the same time were at risk for depression. For those using one of these medications, 7 percent were at risk, and for those taking two of these drugs simultaneously, 9 percent were at risk for depression.

Specific measures of Parasympathetic activity help to differentiate those who are at risk from those who are not. PE is associated with (preclinical) depression. Prolonged or more severe PE can become low SB, which indicates Depression and is a risk indicator

Only the Sympthetics Are Measured

Poor management of Dysautonomia comes largely from the fact that most physicians, including the supposed experts from the Autonomic and Dysautonomia societies, only measure Sympathetic activity. The basis of virtually all medicine, certainly chronic care medicine, is HR, BP, and cardiac output (CO) while at rest. True, the recognized experts test more than at rest. However, their basic assumption is that their patient's Parasympathetic nervous system is so depleted that the test results (which are measuring only total autonomic function, the combination of P&S) are purely Sympathetic in nature. Then they further substantiate their assumptions by comparing them to HR, BP, and CO measurements. Yet BP and CO measures are purely Sympthetic measures, and HR is another total autonomic measure. In effect, their logic and reasoning are circular. They have never measured SW. They do not consider PE as a possibilty, and SE is always considered a primary Dysautonomia.

Some of this may be based on the lack of data, but much of it is based on a not-invented-here syndrome. Through the years, we have tried to work with the recognized experts, but they have developed their own tests which continue to only measure Sympathetic activity or the results of Sympathetic activity, and continue to state that it is not possible to measure Parasympathetic activity directly. What they think are indirect Parasympathetic measures are only measures of total autonomic function; P&S combined. One result of this is that many of the patients that present to P&S monitoring clinics have been turned away from or disillusioned by the recognized expert clinics. Yes, the recognized expert clinics actually say that they cannot, or do not, know how to treat many of these patients.

for suicide.[s] If a patient is prescribed antidepressants or anxiolytics, and after three months, PE is not reduced or relieved, then the patient is not responding to the medication as expected. True, the medication may be masking symptoms, but it is not treating the underlying cause, especially if it is prescribed or has been titrated to high dose. It is strongly recommended that the medication should be switched to an agent to which the patient does respond by demonstrating a reduction in PE. As mentioned above, this is often a switch from SSRIs to tricyclics, typically Nortriptyline (see Anxiety Intervention). Further, as these patients respond to the alternate medication, they often self-wean as the depression is relieved. Reducing the depression also helps to reduce the risk of suicide. Normalizing low SB or PE reduces Depression and also reduces P&S Anxiety. Symptoms of Depression as well as P&S Anxiety typically stem from poor brain perfusion.

As for the other medications that are also known suicide risks, those medications should be titrated so as to not enable or exacerbate PE or low SB. Again, if they do, or if higher doses (as needed) do increase PE, then another agent should be considered that will normalize SB or PE. For example, most beta-blockers, by reducing Sympathetic activity, may increase Parasympathetic activity. If titration of beta-blockers, for example Metoprolol, induces low SB or PE or is recommended to be prescribed for a patient that already demonstrates PE of some sort, then switching to Carvedilol, history dependent, is recommended.

The 26,000-patient study highlights the fact that polypharmacy[t] can lead to depressive symptoms, especially in Anxiety patients, and

---

s   It is also associated with broken heart syndrome, where a surviving spouse from a long-term relationship dies from depression and a suppressed immune system.

t   Polypharmacy is defined as more than one drug prescribed at the same time.

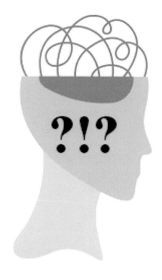

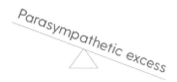

PARASYMPATHETIC
EXCESS WITH SECONDARY
SYMPATHETIC EXCESS

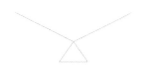

ANXIETY AND DEPRESSION

As discussed above and in our opinion, **P&S Anxiety** is primarily a depression disorder. The hallmark of P&S Anxiety is PE with SE or SW. PE and SW lead to subclinical depression due to poor brain perfusion, and SE is the result of "adrenaline storms" that lead to Anxiety. Primary Anxiety is also associated with SE. Due to poor brain perfusion, the brain is partially "asleep" while you are upright (sitting or standing). This causes many of the symptoms of subclinical depression. This is why antidepressants seem to help, but not totally. So you are prescribed higher doses in the hopes that more is better, or you are prescribed additional medications (there are at least four classes of antidepressants: tricyclics, tetracyclics, SNRIs, and SSRIs) hoping to trample the problem rather than directly addressing the problem. Then, when that does not work, or fully work, they focus on other symptoms, most of which were caused by the overmedication. That is all that most know. They are not taught to look into P&S dysfunction, so that is not a consideration.

that patients and health care providers need to be aware of the risk of depression that comes with all kinds of common prescription drugs. Further, many of these drugs, albeit in reduced dosages, are also available over the counter. Due to their nature of suppressing systems of the body, they may limit blood flow to the brain or limit brain function itself, thereby inducing depression. Examples include: 1) medications to suppress BP or HR to treat hypertension or arrhythmia; or 2) diuretics which reduce blood volume and reduce blood flow to the brain; or 3) anxiolytics or medications to treat ADD or ADHD which reduce or limit brain function; or 4) pain medications to limit pain. This is compounded by the practice of prescribing higher and higher dosages when immediate results are not realized.

The autonomic effects of these medications are to suppress or limit Sympathetic activity, directly or indirectly.[u] While a little limitation helps to normalize SE and prevent disease or disorder, too much Sympathetic suppression leads to low SB or PE. Further, Sympathetic Insufficiency (i.e., SW underlying orthostatic dysfunction) is associated with many of the symptoms of PE. As a result, many may be surprised to learn that these medications may increase their risk of depression, even though they may have nothing to do with mood, depression, or anxiety.

As another example, consider over-the-counter antihistamines. It is well known that temporary, or transient, histaminergic-induced inflammation aids in healing. It is well known that the Sympathetics mediate inflammation. It is also well known that too much or prolonged inflammation and too much or prolonged Sympathetic

---

u   Pain medication is an example of a medication that indirectly reduces Sympathetic activity. It does not directly affect Sympathetic activity; however, it reduces the stress of pain which indirectly reduces Sympathetic activity.

Of course, this is compounded by the lack of restorative sleep. In P&S Anxiety, this symptom is due to gravity. As discussed above, like fainting, once you are laying down (supine) your brain receives the blood it needs to be "awake." So you do not sleep well and the depression deepens.

Unfortunately for patients, this means that antidepressants have been overprescribed (too high dose and too many) and prescribed to far too many people that do not actually need them. Yes, we prescribe antidepressants as part of our recommended therapy program, however we prescribe them at a quarter to a tenth the dose and never for life. Note, when SSRIs were approved by the FDA as antidepressants, the clinical research showed that their efficacy lasted for only forty-five days, on average. Yet we receive patients that have been prescribed these agents for decades. What are these agents doing after forty-five days and what happened to that data?

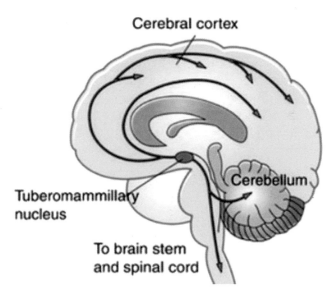

Figure 6: Histaminergic projections originating in the Tuberomammillary Nucleus (TMN) of the Hypothalamus [3] [with permission, 133, Fig. 4,10a]

activity is detrimental. Histaminergic projections in the brain are shown in Figure 6. The Histaminergic system in the brain is phylogenetically old and holds a key position in the regulation of basal body functions, including the sleep-wake cycle, energy and endocrine homeostasis, synaptic plasticity and learning, consciousness, thermoregulation, metabolism, and other life-sustaining functions [60]. Malfunctions in the Histaminergic system are associated with neurological diseases, including Anxiety, Alzheimer's, and Parkinson's, as well as headaches and migraines, difficulty falling asleep, easy arousal, hypertension, vertigo or dizziness, arrhythmia, accelerated HR, difficulty regulating body temperature, nausea, vomiting, abdominal cramps, flushing, nasal congestion, sneezing, difficulty breathing, abnormal menstrual cycle, hives, fatigue, and tissue swelling. Antihistamines are known to have a sedative side-effect. Prolonged antihistamine therapy can lead to depression-like symptoms. Prolonged antihistamine therapy often causes overreaction and stimulates a Histaminergic response to increase inflammation, increasing Sympathetic activity, and possibly exacerbating Anxiety. If antihistamines are needed, as in mast cell activation syndrome (MCAS), the lowest dose should be used in patients with Anxiety or Depression.

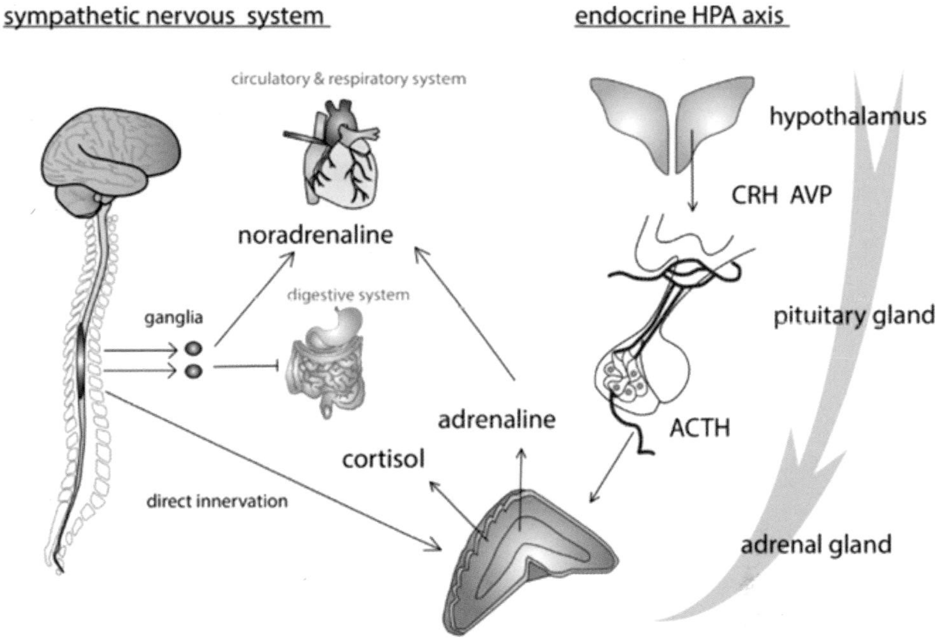

Figure 7: Human stress response pathways operating through the Autonomic Nervous System and the Endocrine System. The Neural and Hormonal signals interact with and complement each other through the regulatory action of the Hypothalamus-Pituitary-Adrenal axis (HPA axis). Abbreviations: ACTH: adreno-corticotropin hormone; AVP: arginine/vasopressin; CRH: cortico-releasing hormone [Open Access, 134].

With the national suicide rate increasing, Depression has become a public health issue. To this end, "Psychopharmacology and Cardiovascular Disease" is an important review in this area [61]. The review's epidemiology shows there are many physiologic and lifestyle risk factors for the development of atherosclerosis with comorbid Depression and Anxiety. These include high lipid levels, hypertension, diabetes, abdominal obesity, physical inactivity, low daily fruit and vegetable consumption, and alcohol over-consumption [62]. There are other psychological factors (besides Depression and Anxiety) as well, such as hostility and type A personality. Granted, the physiologic and lifestyle factors may be the cause of Anxiety and Depression, and these factors are also known to significantly increase risk of cardiovascular disease and negative clinical outcomes.

Hypercortisolism can cause a lower-than-expected response to Corticotropin-Releasing Factor (CRF), increasing CRF [63,64]. Increased CRF increases Adrenocorticotropin (ACTH) secretion, leading to Hypothalamus-Pituitary-Adrenal (HPA) axis overdrive (Figure 7), increasing depression-risk (see Figure 8). Mental (e.g., melancholic or psychotic) and physical (e.g., extreme obesity or chronic pain) stress increases ACTH. ACTH also inhibits most immune functions, and is one of the ways that Depression is known to suppress immune responses, making severe Depression life-threatening. This helps to explain broken heart syndrome.

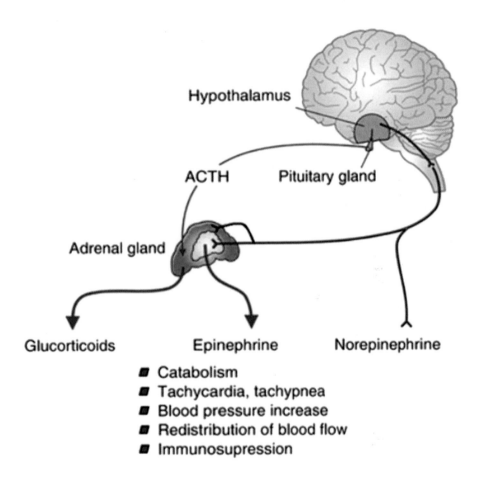

Figure 8: Pituitary release of ACTH activates Adrenal Sympathetic nerves to support defense behavior (fight or flight). [with permission, 133, Fig. 5.12]

Exaggerated platelet reactivity is associated with major depression [65]. Platelets may be activated through several receptor-mediator pathways (see Figure 9) [66]. Serotonin and nitric oxide both play roles in platelet function. Elevated levels of serotonin in the brain help to induce sleep.[v] Too little serotonin in the brain leads to Depression. This is why SSRIs, like Zoloft, help with Depression. SSRIs allow serotonin activity to linger. Nitric oxide helps to establish and maintain endothelial health. Damage to the endothelium stimulates platelet function to minimize blood loss, but it also disrupts blood flow. Under stress, the peripheral vasculature is constricted. Narrowed vessels and turbulent blood flow also promotes platelet function. Nitric oxide helps to relax blood vessels. This may lead to Anxiety. Furthermore, patients with these psychological problems have abnormal HR variability, which can lead to arrhythmias [67] and Anxiety as well. PE is associated with underactive thyroid and other glandular output; of course these are well known to be associated with Depression and Anxiety.

Figure 9 (opposite page): Platelets may be activated through several receptor-mediator pathways. Collagen exposed within the denuded area of vascular endothelium has stimulated platelet activation and adhesion to vessel wall. During activation platelet storage granule contents are extruded and induce irreversible platelet-platelet aggregation and thrombus formation. Activated circulating platelets can be identified by fluorescent-labeled monoclonal antibodies, including PAC1, anti–ligand-induced binding site (LIBS1), GE12, or GA6, V261, and the protein annexin V. Ca++ indicates calcium; PF4, platelet factor 4; β-TG, β-thromboglobulin; ADP, adenosine diphosphate; and 5-HT, serotonin. [66]

---

v   That's why warm milk at bedtime works—serotonin crosses the blood-brain barrier and helps to slow the brain to induce sleep.

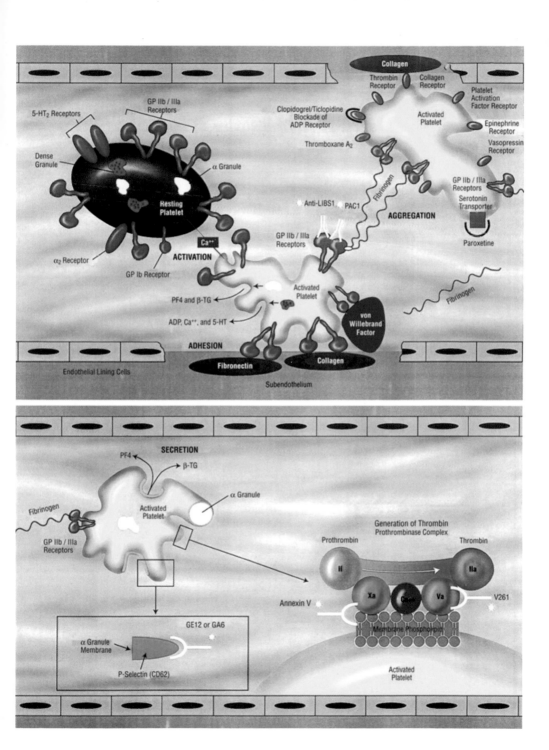

Hypercortisolism and platelet function are parts of the stress response and, if prolonged, these may become atherogenic [68]. Remember, stress responses are meant to be acute (short-term). We are not designed for long-term or chronic stress (including too much food, as in some regions, or all of the psychosocial stress assaulting us hourly). Acute stress has been well studied. Acute stress activates the Sympathetic nervous system, resulting in arrhythmias, endothelial dysfunction, inflammation, and platelet activation [69]. Also, acute stress may affect coronary blood flow, which is mediated by the neuronal nitric oxide synthase (nNOS) pathway [70], which may in turn effect brain perfusion. Inflammation is implicated in coronary plaques and patients who are depressed with multiple cytokines such as C-reactive protein, tumor necrosis factor, interleukin-6, among others [71]. An excessive cytokine response, known as a cytokine "storm," may be exceptionally damaging and is potentially lethal. Extreme inflammation, such as in anaphylaxis, may also be lethal. SE amplifies and exaggerates the acute stress responses (see insert next page) [4].

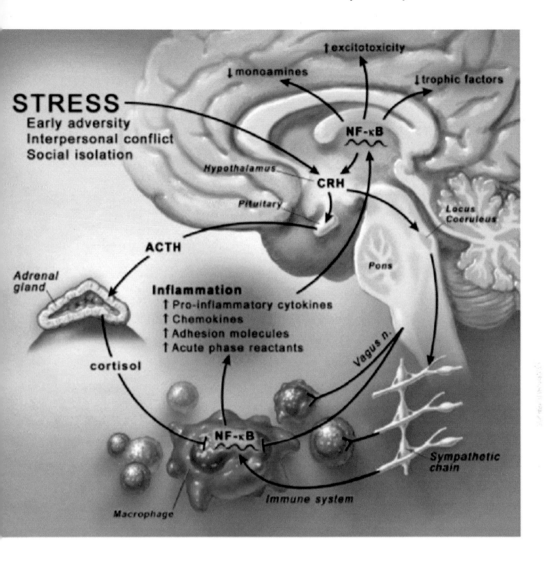

Subjects with Depression have an 80 percent increase in risk for development of new, worsening cardiovascular disease and death from cardiovascular disease [72]. Depression increases the risk of developing cardiovascular disease, and cardiovascular disease can increase the risk of developing Depression. Depression is associated with PE, which may lead to secondary SE, thereby accelerating the stress effects (i.e., endothelial dysfunction, inflammation, and cytokine or platelet activation) leading to the risk increase. PE may also suppress the immune system, effecting cell senescence and apoptosis. Meta-analyses have shown from perspective studies that depression significantly increases the risk of cardiovascular disease. Furthermore, treatment of Depression has been shown to be effective in some studies. It has also been shown that reductions in Depression are associated with modestly reduced coronary heart disease (CHD) risks [73]. A ten-year-follow-up study shows that Anxiety was found to be associated with a 77 percent increased mortality risk and nearly threefold increase risk for CHD [74]. Defense behaviors (stresses) lead to biological responses (see Figure 10) that, when prolonged, are harmful. Chronic diseases, themselves, are possible causes of Anxiety in some patients.

Figure 10 (opposite page): Behavioral and biological aspects of the defense behavior. The sequence of phenomena follows exposure to a novel situation. Strategies are of two types, high or low energy level. The objective is adaptation. If adaptation does not occur, the stress reaction appears, with stimulation of the pituitary-adrenal axis. Illustration by Elysian Creative Studio, www.elysiancreativestudio.com, Lizzy Colombo.

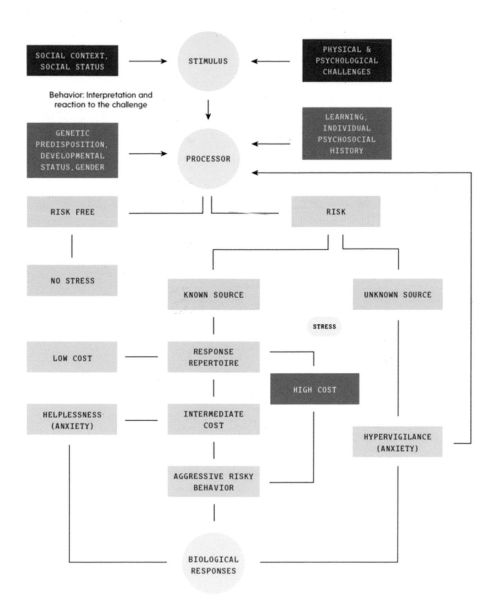

Patients with heart failure who exercise demonstrate a moderate decline in depression symptoms [75]. The presence of anxiety in patients with heart disease was associated with more than twice the risk of CHD and acute MI [76,77], and sudden cardiac death [78]. Patients with Anxiety and Depression were at greater risk of heart disease than patients with either condition alone [79,80] and leads to poor clinical outcomes even in healthy subjects [81]. Causes of Anxiety (i.e., anger) are associated with increase incidences of implantable cardiac defibrillator discharge among cardiac patients [82]. Prolonged, as well as acute, stress is associated with Anxiety. Mental stress, such as (1) intense sporting events, (2) catastrophe, such as earthquake or blizzard, and (3) acute physical activity may increase risk for arrhythmias, myocardial infarction, and sudden cardiac death [81,83,84]. Chronic factors, such as work-related stress, marital dissatisfaction, family stress, psychosocial stresses in general, increase the risk for cardiovascular disease and MACE [81,85,86,87,88].

Figure 11: Acute disease (e.g., myocardial infarction) causes stress responses (e.g., cytokine release) which if prolonged as Anxiety leads to more severe cardiovascular disease. Neural, hormonal, and inflammatory processes indicate sympathetic over-activation contributing to end organ damage, in this case heart failure. Autonomic therapy to establish and maintain SB (e.g., sympatholytics in this case) helps to reduce continued end organ damage. LC = Locus Coeruleus, PVN: Paraventricular Nucleus, RAAS: Renin-Angiotensin-Aldosterone System, RVLM: Rostral Ventrolateral Medulla, SFO: Subfornical Organ, and SON: Supra-Optic Nucleus. Adapted from [77].

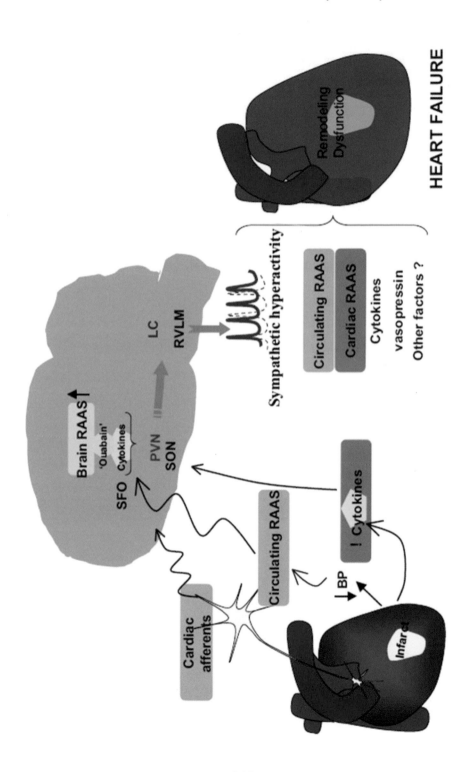

Chronic work stress (low decision latitude and heavy job demands) has been studied extensively. From the field of Neuro-Immunology, it is well known that subordinates are more likely to be ill than are superiors [89]. High psychological demands, lack of social support, and strain were associated with increased risk for heart disease; whereas, effort, reward and balance, job sensitivity, and long working hours were not related [86]. Risk increases with all types of stress in comparison with age-matched controls [90]. Risk triples with prolonged stress as demonstrated in a five-year follow-up study, even when adjusting for background and health related factors [91]. The INTERHEART Study demonstrated that psychosocial stress increases risk of MI by more than a factor of 2 [90]. Biological stress (see Figure 10) exerts a complex interaction of hemodynamic, inflammatory, neural, humeral, and hemostatic changes that account for the increased incidence of disease (increase morbidity risk) as exemplified by myocardial infarction and coronary atherosclerosis (see Figure 11) [92].

Inflammation is also an important response to stress. Prolonged stress, as in Anxiety, prolongs inflammation, which also increases morbidity and mortality risk through increases in many oxidative-induced diseases such as coronary atherosclerosis. Again, inflammation is mediated by the Sympathetics. There are many inflammatory markers that have been followed and studied including CRP, IL-6, and TNF-alpha. Also, fibrinogen as an acute phase reaction has hemostatic and inflammatory properties. Fibrinogen has been a risk factor for CHD, stroke, and vascular mortality [93].

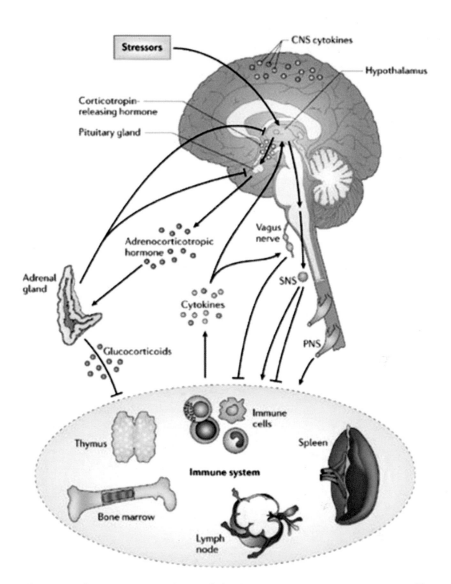

Figure: Inflammatory markers of the immune system, components affected by inflammation due to stress as mediated through the P&S nervous systems and hormone system. Chronic disease may lead to Anxiety. See insert above [with permission 133].

PTSD is strongly associated with other psychiatric disorders, including Anxiety and Depression, which have been shown to predict cardiovascular events [94,95]; associated markers include: inflammatory markers (i.e., tumor necrosis factor, interleukins, von Willebrand factor antigen, clotting factor VII, and fibrinogen) [96,97]. Also, PTSD is associated with high cortisol levels and peripheral adrenergic activity [98]. Sympathetic overactivity (secondary to PE in response to stress, in our experience) increases norepinephrine levels and pro-inflammatory and pro-coagulant changes which contribute to ongoing inflammation and hypercoagulable states in PTSD. This can promote clot formation and plaque ruptures and myocardial infarction. There is also low resting vagal tone (high SB) in PTSD and, in this case, the protective mechanism or braking mechanism is being nullified. Pro-inflammatory toxins produced by immune cells can exert adverse effects on the Parasympathetics [99,100].

All in all, Anxiety resulting in chronic mental stress is an extreme risk factor, including mortality. The various morbidity risks, including endocrine, autoimmune, metabolic, cardiovascular, and psychiatric changes, increase or lead to mortality risks, such as from obesity leading to metabolic syndrome, and insulin resistance, leading to diabetes, and eventually cardiovascular disease. This is significantly compounded by the P&S dysfunctions that underlie ALDs. Anxiety is predictive of life-threatening events (e.g., MACE) [101]. It doubles MACE risk [102]. The combination of disease and Anxiety triples risk for additional clinical events, including recurrent cardiac events [103]. Therapy to relieve Anxiety is associated with a 28 percent reduction in mortality in comparison with controls

Acute stress prepares biological organisms (including you) for fight-or-flight defense mechanisms. With acute stress, both (1) norepinephrine (noradrenaline, the adrenaline found in nerves) is released from the Sympathetic fibers and (2) adrenalin (epinephrine, the hormone) from the adrenal glands. Norepinephrine stimulates alpha-1 and beta-1 Sympathetic receptors and epinephrine stimulates alpha-2 and beta-2 Sympathetic receptors. The alpha receptors help to control the arteries and veins and the beta receptors help to control the heart and lungs. Catecholamines[w] are rapidly cleared to keep the response short. During acute stress with a defense reaction, there is Sympathetic activation of most of the organs in the body. In addition, cortisol is secreted to help buffer the stresses involved in the fight or flight reaction, and the Renin-Angiotensin system is activated to increase BP. The Renin-Angiotensin system is one of the pathways that controls BP, both through the hormone Angiotensin and a portion of the Sympathetic nervous system stimulated by Renin. There is also withdrawal of Parasympathetic activity which contributes to increases in HR along with Sympathetic activation. The Hypothalamic-Pituitary-Adrenal Axis (see Figure 7) is very important in coordinating the stress response. Steroids (e.g., glucocorticoids) are major components of the stress systems and affect many different systems. They can attenuate inflammation, cellular proliferation, and tissue repair processes. All of these responses are designed to be short-term.

As these responses persist and become long-term, such as with Anxiety, various endocrine, autoimmune, metabolic, cardiovascular, and psychiatric changes occur which increases morbidity and mortality risks, decreasing quality of life and longevity, respectively. These include stress-induced hypercortisolism and central obesity, which is a component of metabolic syndrome. Visceral

---

w Norepinephrine (noradrenaline) and adrenalin (epinephrine) are collectively known as catecholamines.

from a two-year follow-up [78]. Therapy to balance the P&S with supplements and lifestyle changes relieves Anxiety in addition to pharmaceutical therapy, is recommended, history dependent. Appropriate antioxidant balance to help reestablish P&S balance to treat underlying oxidative stress is a key to controlling ALDs.

NEUROFEEDBACK (edited by Richard Lill, LCSW)

As you know, the electroencephalogram (EEG) is a recording of the electrical activity of the brain and is largely comprised of four clinical frequencies that have been associated with certain (normal) and essential daily activities, such as: sleep, relaxed attention, and hyper-attention. The different frequencies are labeled [104]: Alpha, Beta, Delta, and Theta. Each of these brainwave frequencies are always present to some degree in different parts of the brain [105].

EEG biofeedback (also known as neurofeedback[x]) has been in use as a clinical intervention for well over thirty years. It has been stated in conference that 298 of 315 major studies have demonstrated success. Yet neurofeedback remains underutilized. One reason for this has been the difficulty in obtaining quantitative measures of clinical outcomes. P&S monitoring, however, provides quantitative measures. It is well known that the individual P&S branches are associated with the different frequencies and different portions of the brain. There is substantial evidence exists for its efficacy in treating ADHD.

Cortical plasticity can be changed with computer brain interface (CBI) techniques. CBI provides visual or auditory feedback to

---

x   This is not HRV-biofeedback

obesity from stress is a result of chronic cortisol elevations. Chronic stress from Anxiety increases appetite, Sympathetic activation, and Hypothalamic-Pituitary-Adrenal Axis activity which further increases cortisol. This leads to more visceral obesity, metabolic syndrome, and insulin resistance, and eventually diabetes. Endothelial damage and atherosclerosis with its inherent risk of cardiovascular events and mortality can ensue. Supplement and lifestyle changes along with pharmacology and appropriate antioxidant balance are very important in controlling this.

NEUROFEEDBACK (edited by Richard Lill, LCSW)

When our brainwaves are not operating optimally, it results in unwanted thoughts, feelings, and behaviors, including Anxiety. Neurofeedback can painlessly correct the brainwaves to alleviate those behaviors and feelings. It helps you to learn how to modify your brainwave patterns on demand, calming the mind, reducing Anxiety, impulse behaviors, and depression, and improving attention.

Neurofeedback is also known as electroencephalogram (EEG) Biofeedback. It is currently being used for performance enhancement, mental focus, and tranquility. Neurofeedback is reported to have positive treatment outcomes or normalizing trends in various disorders, including children with autism, patients with ADHD, and in studies designed to enhance cognitive and musical performance. Neurofeedback is based on the neuroscience of the EEG. The EEG is a recording of the electrical activity of the brain. A study of the EEG demonstrates certain waveforms at certain frequencies are associated with certain (normal) and essential daily activities, such as: sleep, relaxed attention, and hyper-attention. The different types of brainwaves that have been identified and correlated are:

alter neural activity. Lasting changes in cortical plasticity have been detected following neurofeedback. Neurofeedback is a relatively user-friendly method to operantly condition brain activity. It has been shown to be able to induce a specific increase of functional connectivity within the alertness/salience network (dorsal anterior and mid cingulate), when compared with a sham control group [106]. Neurofeedback is thought to indirectly modify behavior by changing neuronal activation or connectivity patterns in the Central Nervous System via operant conditioning. Neurofeedback has been shown to be able to reshape neural activity, as measured by EEG frequency components [107] and fMRI [108,109]. Positive outcomes have been reported for neurofeedback for Anxiety [110,111], children with autism [112,113], ADHD [114,115,116], Depression [117], substance abuse [118,119,120], PTSD [121,122], epilepsy [123], and obsessive-compulsive disorder [124], and it also has positive outcomes in performance enhancement [125], cognitive and musical performance [126], and motor learning [127].

Neurofeedback is an operant conditioning technique used to reinforce or inhibit specific forms of EEG activity [128,129]. It is a therapeutic method designed to train the mind and body to act in a more optimal way in order to improve emotional, cognitive, physical, and behavioral experiences [130]. Neuropathology research has shown that turning abnormal rhythms and frequencies (based on Quantitative-EEG, or QEEG^y) into normal (or relatively normal) rhythms and frequencies, thereby turning abnormal psychological states into normal ones [131].

---

y As a comprehensive assessment tool endorsed by both the American Psychological Association and the International Society for Neurofeedback and Research, QEEG is used by qualified health care professionals to objectively and scientifically evaluate a patient's brainwave function to determine whether brainwave patterns are abnormal and, if so, where and why these abnormalities occur.

- Alpha—waveforms associated generally with a state of relaxation (8–12 Hz)
- Beta—the fastest of the waveforms correlated, which represent a state of mental, intellectual activity, outward focused attention (12–35 Hz). The lower end of this frequency band (e.g., Sensorimotor Rhythm or SMR) corresponds to a state of relaxed attentiveness (12–15 Hz);
  ◊ the hyper-state of high-frequency beta brainwaves is as high as 35 Hz;
- Delta—the slowest of the waveforms correlated, which are associated with deep restorative sleep (0.5–3.5 Hz);
- Theta—waveforms represent a deeply relaxed, daydreaming state (4-8 Hz).

In neurofeedback therapy, also known as training, neural activity is recorded from scalp electrodes and fed back in real time to subjects in a readily understood, visual format (simple computer games). Neurofeedback-associated EEG changes have been correlated with changes in various functional outcomes, including cortico-motor excitability (motor learning), memory, cognition, sleep, and mood, as well as increases in effect regulation and executive function, sustained attention, and working memory. By challenging the brain, much as the body is challenged in physical exercise, the brain may be helped to learn to function better.

As an example, if someone is experiencing acute Anxiety, an excess of high-frequency beta brainwaves may be present in a certain brain region, or it may be a result of an abnormal amount (too much or too little) of Alpha brainwaves in the Parietal regions of the brain (toward the back of the cortex) that are associated with the control of emotions. Neurofeedback therapy relieves these excessive frequencies to relieve the Anxiety in a video game–like format.

During amplitude training, protocols are decided based on the QEEG or Mini-Map, which utilizes three points down the middle of the scalp (front to back). The Mini-map helps to determine whether the client's brain is under-aroused or over-aroused. When exploring the Mini-Map, in addition to history and symptoms, it may be determined that the individual's brain would meet criteria for an Unstable Arousal. Unstable Arousal is typically found with patients who experience migraines, seizures, head injuries, and Bipolar Disorder, or Disordered Arousal. Disordered Arousal is typical of patients with autism and Developmental Trauma. History becomes imperative with these patients at this point in order to ensure success in training.

After evaluation, a determination is made as to which protocol is most commonly going to reward the Sensory Motor Rhythm (SMR) Beta or Alpha rhythm. At this time, the practitioner works to find the placement and frequency that works best for the patient, taking direction from the Mini-Map or QEEG results.

Alpha-Training: Based on the initial evaluation it may be determined that an individual may have low Alpha activity which seems to be best measured toward the back of the scalp. In cases of low-Alpha, it may be decided to utilize neurofeedback to increase Alpha brain waves. This may be done by rewarding Alpha while inhibiting the other brainwaves. Overarousal has also been recognized in individuals who have Alpha that is too high as well, which is why the initial evaluations are important in determining what the individual would benefit from.

Sensory Motor Rhythm (SMR, 12–15 Hz) Beta (15–18 Hz) Training: This is a common form of training where the reward frequencies will be 12–15 on the right side to decrease arousal

Experience indicates that after fifteen sessions of neurofeedback, patients may experience long-term benefits (positive changes) in personality variables. Some may take more sessions and some may take less; the important point is your openness to change. Alpha-Theta Training is one form of neurofeedback, and is believed be associated with an increase in beta-endorphin levels related to reduced stress.

Neurofeedback may help to:

- *Improve sleep patterns.* More efficient sleep is associated with being more alert during the day, reduced anxiety and depression, and reduced migraine or chronic pain.
- *Improve focus and enable more attention,* as measured by how well one persists even at an unwanted task.
- *Improve the management of emotions.* Emotions, like perceptions, are real to the individual, but the brain has a lot to say about how the individual will respond to emotions, how the individual will feel and react. Out-of-control emotions are not good, but one can be trained. No emotions (i.e., a lack of empathy) is not good, but one can be trained.
- *Reduce some forms of seizures* by reorganizing the brain to bypass the circuits that generate seizure.
- *Normalize traumatic brain injury, including concussion and stroke,* by reorganizing the brain to bypass the injured circuits.
- *Train (retrain) the brain in autism* to function better and possibly engage the circuits that are being bypassed.

Before the training begins, specific objectives are established by you or in cooperation with your loved ones. In order to reach a specific objective, the training usually continues for a specific number of sessions. If there is a loss of optimal training effect after completion, due to stresses in life, a few booster sessions may be recommended. However, just as concert pianists practice more than the rest, rather than less, neurofeedback training can be used without limit to enhance performance.

and 15–18 on the left side to increase arousal. In individuals who suffer from anxiety or an over aroused brain it is common practice to work on the right hemisphere, which should alleviate any anxiety symptoms. Success in any neurofeedback training will likely be determined by the client over the following twenty-four to forty-eight hours and any change will fade away. Training includes approximately thirty SMR/Beta training sessions (depending on severity) of fifty minutes each over a two-month period. SMR/Beta neurofeedback training focuses on the Sensory Motor Strip and has been demonstrated to reduce Anxiety, improve aspects of personality, and decrease stress-related and blood-based beta-endorphins [132].

In SMR/Beta-training (visual, relaxed attention), the suppressed frequencies were Delta (2–5 Hz), Theta (5–8 Hz), and high Beta (18–30 Hz). Thresholds were adjusted in a way that if the participant maintained the reinforcement band above the threshold for 80 percent of the time for a duration of at least 0.5 second, and the suppressed band under the threshold for 20 percent of the time, feedback was received. Whenever participants could maintain the reinforcement band's above the threshold for 90 percent of the time during two continuous trials, the threshold was changed automatically so that it was closer to the optimal threshold.

Alpha-Theta or Alpha Neurofeedback Training includes approximately thirty Sensory Motor Rhythm (SMR) training sessions (depending on severity) of twenty minutes each over a two-month period. Alpha-theta neurofeedback training focuses on the Parietal brain cortex area, and has been demonstrated to improve mood, personality inventory scales, ability to focus, and ability to processes information, with demonstrated benefits for patients with PTSD and Addiction, and individuals training for Peak Performance. Neurofeedback could be effective in helping adolescents.

This "peak performance training" may be of interest to many, including professional athletes, corporate executives, and performing artists.

Example fMRI brain map, frequency composites for Normal, ADHD, Depression, Anxiety, and migraine (in order from left to right).

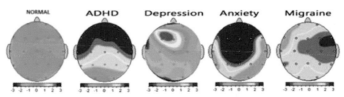

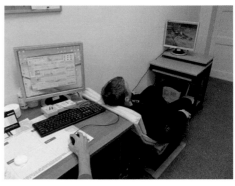

Neurofeedback electrode placement sites to measure the waveforms that are being trained (left) with corresponding cortical areas presented (right).

Therapy is like playing video games with your brain.

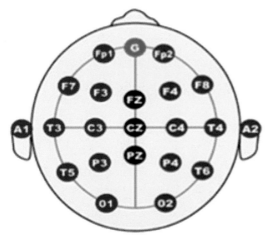

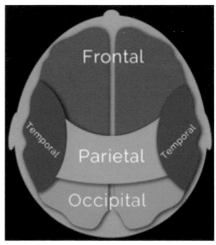

In the Alpha-Theta training (audio, eyes closed, relaxed attention), the reinforcement band was 5–8 Hz (Theta) and 8–12 Hz (Alpha). The initial sessions were used to train patients to decrease Alpha levels that were above 12 mV (peak to peak), while augmenting Theta, until the Alpha amplitude dropped to function better. Based on neuropathology, this method has shown evidence of turning abnormal rhythms and frequencies (based on Quantitative-EEG[z]) into normal (or relatively normal) rhythms and frequencies, thereby turning abnormal psychological states into normal ones. Especially if comorbid problems are present, it is critical that accurate assessment is made prior to neurofeedback treatment in order to determine excesses and deficiencies of given brainwave frequencies, and where these abnormalities may occur in the brain, taking into consideration comorbidities to ensure individualized patient treatment.

---

z   As a comprehensive assessment tool endorsed by both the American Psychological Association and the International Society for Neurofeedback and Research, QEEG is used by qualified health care professionals to objectively and scientifically evaluate a patient's brainwave function to determine whether brainwave patterns are abnormal and, if so, where and why these abnormalities occur.

Before Treatment

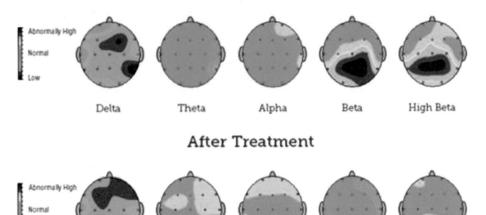

After Treatment

An example of the effects of neurofeedback training on an ADHD patient. Depicted are the fMRI brain maps of the different individual EEG frequencies. Alpha-Theta training therapy normalized the higher (hyper) frequency Beta waveforms associated with ADHD (reduced the reds and yellows) and enhanced the lower (calmer) frequency Alpha and Theta waveforms (increased the greens). This teenage patient is less hyper and reactive, and better able to focus and concentrate. Shortly after therapy, this patient was weaned from the stimulants (Adderall) he was prescribed. He required four follow-up sessions, and has been therapy free for over two years. (Blue = under-activity, Green = normal, Red = overactivity).

BEST TO AVOID

The primary goal of therapy in P&S Anxiety or in ALD cases is to stimulate the brain by normalizing brain (and coronary) perfusion pressures, rather than chemically, such as with Ritalin or Adderall. Establishing proper daily hydration and proper P&S Balance, both at rest and in response to challenge, is the plan to achieve the goal of normalizing brain perfusion. To establish P&S balance, low-dose therapy is recommended. Moderate to high doses will cause more symptoms by pushing the balance too far to the opposite branch. Low and slow therapy also recognizes that establishing P&S balance cannot be rushed. Titrating therapy too fast will also push the balance too far. Again, the P&S is like a pendulum. Hitting a pendulum with a hammer to correct it only knocks it off its hinge and makes matters worse. It takes small, gentle nudges over time to correct. As an older, wise medical school professor told us, "Your patient had to go up and over a mountain to arrive at the place they were in when they first presented. They will have to climb up and over that same mountain if they are to return to the state they were in to begin with. There is no tunneling to create shortcuts."

The main reason for low and slow therapy is the fact that the P&S nervous systems affect the whole body, so any therapy will affect the whole body, including the other organs and systems.

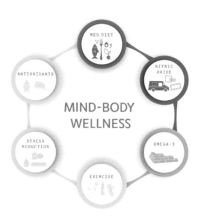

Attempting to normalize one organ or system will undoubtedly affect other organs or systems, and not always positively. To this end, we recommend minimal pharmaceutical therapy to do as much acceleration of therapy as possible without overcorrecting the balance. This, plus the fact that there are very limited approved choices for pharmaceutical therapies, and therefore, therapies are typically used off-label, we have

BEST TO AVOID

Patients with Dysautonomia tend to be sensitive to many things. You often know best when you tend to be sensitive to what and have developed means of avoiding or living with them. This can include temperature (heat or cold), chemicals (e.g., food, drink, prescription and over-the-counter medications, lotions, oils, powders, etc.). Some of the most common avoidances are heat and alcohol. Heat represents stress. In general, stress is to be avoided until the P&S nervous systems are retrained to accept little stresses, then the bigger ones may be reintroduced. Often, moderate to heavy exercise is enjoyed with patients with Dysautonomia, but they then suffer once it is finished. This is because the exercise helps to circulate blood to the heart and brain. You are able to think more clearly and feel more energized. However, you are actually doing yourself a disservice in the long run. Don't worry, you will return to the heavier exercise, but until the nervous system is retrained to accept little stresses without "crashing," you should stay away from the bigger stresses. Food can be a stress. We were not created to have a restaurant on every street corner, nor indulge in large meals. To this end, large, heavy meals should be avoided, for not only is that much food stressful, but the obesity that may ensue is also a stress. In fact, for many with Dysautonomia, most things have become a stress, and excesses and extremes should be avoided while your nervous systems are returning to balance. All in all, while under therapy, you must listen to your body while you are returning to balance.

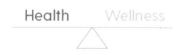

developed a more natural approach. Our approach uses supplements and lifestyle modifications. The basis for this approach is to restore blood volume with proper daily hydration (48 ounces to 64 ounces of water a day including reducing diuretics and reducing consumption of alcohol, caffinated, and sugar drinks; including artifical sugars), and to relieve oxidative stress with therapeutic doses of direct and indirect antioxidants, including r-ALA, CoEnzyme Q10, low and slow exercise, a diet high in fresh fruits and vegetables, and Stress reduction, as direct **antioxidants**, and nitric oxide boosters and omega-3 fatty acids, as indirect antioxidants. This formula not only helps you to make your patients healthy, it will help you to make them well.

DISEASE &
DISORDER

Antioxidants Oxidants

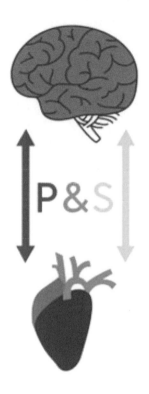

REFERENCES

1. https://www.cdc.gov/ Accessed 4 July 2019

2. Nepon J, Belik SL, Bolton J, Sareen J. The relationship between anxiety disorders and suicide attempts: findings from the National Epidemiologic Survey on Alcohol and Related Conditions. *Depress Anxiety.* 2010;27(9):791–8.

3. DePace NL, Colombo J. *Autonomic and Mitochondrial Dysfunction in Clinical Diseases: Diagnostic, Prevention, and Therapy.* Springer Science + Business Media, New York, 2019.

4. Tobias H, Vinitsky A, Bulgarelli RJ, Ghosh-Dastidar S, Colombo J. Autonomic nervous system monitoring of patients with excess parasympathetic responses to sympathetic challenges—clinical observations. *US Neurology.* 2010; 5(2): 62–66.

5. Bystritsky A, Khalsa SS, Cameron ME, Schiffman J. Current diagnosis and treatment of anxiety disorders. *P T.* 2013;38(1):30–57.

6. Bouayed J, Rammal H, Soulimani R. Oxidative stress and anxiety: relationship and cellular pathways. *Oxid Med Cell Longev.* 2009;2(2):63–7.

7. Salim S. Oxidative stress and psychological disorders. *Curr Neuropharmacol.* 2014;12(2):140–47.

8. Hassan W, Silva CE, Mohammadzai IU, da Rocha JB, J LF. Association of oxidative stress to the genesis of anxiety: implications for possible therapeutic interventions. *Curr Neuropharmacol.* 2014;12(2):120–39.

9. Čeprnja M., Vuletić V. Oxidative Stress and Anxiety Disorder. In: Dietrich-Muszalska A., Chauhan V., Grignon S. (eds) *Studies on Psychiatric Disorders. Oxidative Stress in Applied Basic Research and Clinical Practice.* Humana Press, New York, 2015.

10. Fedoce ADG, Ferreira F, Bota RG, Bonet-Costa V, Sun PY, Davies KJA. The role of oxidative stress in anxiety disorder: cause or consequence? *Free Radic Res.* 2018 Jul;52(7):737–50. doi: 10.1080/10715762.2018.1475733. Epub 2018 Jun 4.

11. Murray GL and Colombo J. (R)Alpha Lipoic Acid is a Safe, Effective Pharmacologic Therapy of Chronic Orthostatic Hypotension Associated with Low Sympathetic Tone. *Int J Angiol.* In Print, 2018.

12. Vinik AI, Maser RE, Nakave AA. Diabetic cardiovascular autonomic nerve dysfunction. *US Endocrine Disease.* 2007; Dec: 2–9.

13. Vinik A, Ziegler D. Diabetic cardiovascular autonomic neuropathy. *Circulation.* 2007; 115: 387–97.

14. Akselrod S, Gordon S, Ubel FA, Shannon DC, Berger AC, Cohen RJ. "Power spectrum analysis of heart rate fluctuations: a quantitative probe of beat-to- beat cardiovascular control." *Science*, 1981; 213:213–20.

15. Akselrod S, Gordon D, Madwed JB, Snidman NC, Shannon DC, Cohen RJ. Hemodynamic regulation: investigation by spectra analysis. *Am J Physiol* 1985; 249:H867–75.

16. Akselrod S, Eliash S, Oz O, Cohen S. Hemodynamic regulation in SHR: investigation by spectral analysis. *Am J Physiol* 1987; 253:II176–83.

17. Akselrod S: Spectral analysis of fluctuations in cardiovascular parameters: a quantitative tool for the investigation of autonomic control. Trends Pharmacol Sci 1988; 9: 6–9.

18. Goldberger JJ, Arora R, Buckley U, Shivkumar K. Autonomic Nervous System Dysfunction: JACC Focus Seminar. *J Am Coll Cardiol*. 2019 Mar 19;73(10):1189–1206. doi: 10.1016/j.jacc.2018.12.064.

19. Bloomfield DM, Kaufman ES, Bigger JT Jr, Fleiss J, Rolnitzky L, Steinman R. Passive head-up tilt and actively standing up produce similar overall changes in autonomic balance. *Am Heart J*. 1997 Aug;134 (2 Pt 1):316–20.

20. Wikipedia contributors. "Da Costa syndrome." Wikipedia, 25 Feb. 2020. Web. 1 Apr. 2020.

21. "Da Costa syndrome". www.whonamedit.com. Retrieved 2007-12-18.

22. National Research Council; Committee on Veterans' Compensation for Posttraumatic Stress Disorder (2007). *PTSD Compensation and Military Service: Progress and Promise*. Washington, D.C: National Academies Press. p. 35. Retrieved 2008-05-26. Being able to attribute soldier's heart to a physical cause provided an "honorable solution" to all vested parties, as it left the self-respect of the soldier intact and it kept military authorities from having to explain the "psychological breakdowns in previously brave soldiers" or to account for "such troublesome issues as cowardice, low unit morale, poor leadership, or the meaning of the war effort itself" (Van der Kolk et al., as cited in Lasiuk, 2006).

23. Edmund D., MD Pellegrino; Caplan, Arthur L.; Mccartney, James Elvins; Dominic A. Sisti (2004). *Health, Disease, and Illness: Concepts in Medicine*. Washington, D.C: Georgetown University Press. p. 165.

24. World Health Organization (1992). *Icd-10: The Icd-10 Classification of Mental and Behavioural Disorders: Clinical Descriptions and Diagnostic Guidelines*. Geneva: World Health Organization. p. 168.

25. Goetz, C.G. (1993). Turner C.M.; Aminoff M.J. (eds.). *Handbook of Clinical Neurology*. B.V.: Elsevier Science Publishers. pp. 429–47.

26. Mackenzie, Sir James; R. M. Wilson; Philip Hamill; Alexander Morrison; O. Leyton; Florence A. Stoney (1916-01-18). "Discussions On The Soldier's Heart". *Proceedings of the Royal Society of Medicine, Therapeutical and Pharmacological Section*. 9: 27–60.

27. Da Costa, Jacob Medes (January 1871). "On irritable heart; a clinical study of a form of functional cardiac disorder and its consequences". *The American Journal of the Medical Sciences* (61): 18–52.

References

28. "2008 ICD-9-CM Diagnosis 306.* - Physiological malfunction arising from mental factors". 2008 ICD-9-CM Volume 1 Diagnosis Codes. Retrieved 2008-05-26. Neurocirculatory asthenia is most typically seen as a form of anxiety disorder.

29. "Dorlands Medical Dictionary:Da Costa syndrome". Retrieved 2008-05-26.

30. "Neurasthenia". Rare Disease Database. National Organization for Rare Disorders, Inc. 2005. Retrieved 2008-05-28.

31. Paul Wood, MD (1941-05-24). "Da Costa syndrome (or Effort Syndrome). Lecture I". Lectures to the Royal College of Physicians of London. *British Medical Journal.* pp. 1(4194): 767–772. Retrieved 2008-05-28.

32. Cohen ME, White PD (November 1, 1951). "Life situations, emotions, and neurocirculatory asthenia (anxiety neurosis, neurasthenia, effort syndrome)". *Psychosomatic Medicine.* 13 (6): 335–57. doi:10.1097/00006842-195111000-00001.

33. Paul O (1987). "Da Costa syndrome or neurocirculatory asthenia". *British Heart Journal.* 58 (4): 306–15. doi:10.1136/hrt.58.4.306.

34. DePace NL, Colombo J. *Fatigue & Dysautonomia Chronic or Persistent, What's the Difference? The Mind-Body Wellness Program,* Skyhorse, In Print.

35. Low et al., Postural Tachycardia Syndrome (POTS), *Journal of Cardiovascular Electrophysiology.* 20(3):352–8 (2009).

36. Online Mendelian Inheritance in Man (OMIM) Orthostatic Intolerance -604715

37. http://www.clevelandclinicmeded.com/medicalpubs/diseasemanagement/psychiatry-psychology/anxiety-disorder/ (Jess Rowney, Teresa Hermida, Donald Malone, 2010): Definition and etiology Accessed 4 July 2019

38. Weissman M, Wickramaratne P, Nomura Y, et al: Offspring of depressed parents: 20 years later. *Am J Psychiatry.* 2006, 163: 1001–8.

39. https://www.psychiatry.org/psychiatrists/practice/dsm accessed 4 July 2019

40. Colombo J, Arora RR, DePace NL, Vinik AI. *Clinical Autonomic Dysfunction: Measurement, Indications, Therapies, and Outcomes.* Springer Science + Business Media, New York, 2014.

41. Tobias H, Vinitsky A, Bulgarelli RJ, Ghosh-Dastidar S, Colombo J. Autonomic nervous system monitoring of patients with excess Parasympathetic responses to Sympathetic challenges—clinical observations. *US Neurology.* 2010; 5(2): 62–6.

42. Colombo J, Murray GL, Pinales JM, Acosta C, Lill R, Friedman MJ and DePace NL. Parasympathetic and Sympathetic Nervous System Monitoring and Anxiety-Like Symptoms: Improved Differentiation and Improved Outcomes. *Cardio Open.* 06 April 2020; 5(1): 19–25.

43. DePace NL, Acosta CR, and Colombo J. Oral vasoactive medications: A review of Midodrine, Droxidopa, and Pseudoephedrine as applied to orthostatic dysfunction. *Clin Pharmacol Ther.* Submitted. June 2020.

44. Williams KA, Patel H. Healthy plant-based diet: What does it really mean?. *JACC*. 2017; 70(4): 423–5.

45. Grases G, Colom MA, Fernandez RA, Costa-Bauzá A, Grases F. Evidence of higher oxidative status in depression and anxiety. *Oxid Med Cell Longev*. 2014;2014:430216. doi: 10.1155/2014/430216. Epub 2014 Apr 29.

46. McIntyre RS, Soczynska JK, Lewis GF, MacQueen GM, Konarski JZ, Kennedy SH. Managing psychiatric disorders with antidiabetic agents: translational research and treatment opportunities. *Expert Opin Pharmacother*. 2006 Jul;7(10):1305–21.

47. See Figure 187 and the "Homocysteine" section, references 1270 and 1558 of [3].

48. Nabavi SM, Daglia M, Braidy N, Nabavi SF. Natural products, micronutrients, and nutraceuticals for the treatment of depression: A short review. *Nutr Neurosci*. 2017 Apr; 20(3):180–94. doi: 10.1080/1028415X.2015.1103461. Epub 2015 Nov 27.

49. Kinrys G, Coleman E, Rothstein E. Natural remedies for anxiety disorders: potential use and clinical applications. *Depress Anxiety*. 2009;26(3):259-65. doi: 10.1002/da.20460.

50. Lakhan SE, Vieira KF. Nutritional and herbal supplements for anxiety and anxiety-related disorders: systematic review. *Nutr J*. 2010 Oct 7;9:42. doi: 10.1186/1475-2891-9-42.

51. Smaga I, Niedzielska E, Gawlik M, Moniczewski A, Krzek J, Przegaliński E, Pera J, Filip M. Oxidative stress as an etiological factor and a potential treatment target of psychiatric disorders. Part 2. Depression, anxiety, schizophrenia and autism. *Pharmacol Rep*. 2015 Jun;67(3):569-80. doi: 10.1016/j.pharep.2014.12.015. Epub 2015 Jan 5.

52. Müller CP, Reichel M, Mühle C, Rhein C, Gulbins E, Kornhuber J. Brain membrane lipids in major depression and anxiety disorders. *Biochim Biophys Acta*. 2015 Aug;1851(8):1052–65. doi: 10.1016/j.bbalip.2014.12.014. Epub 2014 Dec 24.

53. Hennebelle M, Champeil-Potokar G, Lavialle M, Vancassel S, Denis I. Omega-3 polyunsaturated fatty acids and chronic stress-induced modulations of glutamatergic neurotransmission in the hippocampus. *Nutr Rev*. 2014 Feb;72(2):99–112. doi: 10.1111/nure.12088. Epub 2014 Jan 13.

54. Appleton KM, Sallis HM, Perry R, Ness AR, Churchill R. ω-3 Fatty acids for major depressive disorder in adults: an abridged Cochrane. *BMJ Open*. 2016 Mar 2;6(3):e010172. doi: 10.1136/bmjopen-2015-010172.

55. Vesco AT, Lehmann J, Gracious BL, Arnold LE, Young AS, Fristad MA. Omega-3 Supplementation for Psychotic Mania and Comorbid Anxiety in Children. *J Child Adolesc Psychopharmacol*. 2015 Sep;25(7):526–34. doi: 10.1089/cap.2013.0141. Epub 2015 Aug 19.

56. Kumar A, Chanana P. Role of Nitric Oxide in Stress-Induced Anxiety: From Pathophysiology to Therapeutic Target. *Vitam Horm*. 2017;103:147-167. doi: 10.1016/bs.vh.2016.09.004. Epub 2016 Dec 2.

References

57. Gulati K, Rai N, Ray A. Nitric Oxide and Anxiety. *Vitam Horm.* 2017;103:169–92. doi: 10.1016/bs.vh.2016.09.001. Epub 2016 Oct 31.

58. Grijalva CG, Biaggioni I, Griffin MR, Shibao CA. Fludrocortisone Is Associated With a Higher Risk of All-Cause Hospitalizations Compared With Midodrine in Patients With Orthostatic Hypotension. *J Am Heart Assoc.* 2017 Oct 12;6(10). pii: e006848. doi: 10.1161/JAHA.117.006848.

59. Qato DM, Ozenberger K, Olfson M. Prevalence of Prescription Medications With Depression as a Potential Adverse Effect Among Adults in the United States. *JAMA.* 2018; 319(22): 2289. DOI: 10.1001/jama.2018.6741.

60. Haas H and Panula P. The role of histamine and the tuberomammillary nucleus in the nervous system. *Nat Rev Neurosci.* 2003; 4: 121–30.

61. Piña IL, Di Palo KE, Ventura HO. Psychopharmacology and Cardiovascular Disease. *JACC.* 2018; 71(20): 2346–59.

62. American Heart Association Nutrition Committee, Lichtenstein AH, Appel LJ, Brands M, Carnethon M, Daniels S, Franch HA, Franklin B, Kris-Etherton P, Harris WS, Howard B, Karanja N, Lefevre M, Rudel L, Sacks F, Van Horn L, Winston M, Wylie-Rosett J. *Diet and lifestyle recommendations revision 2006: a scientific statement from the American Heart Association Nutrition Committee. Circulation.* 2006 Jul 4;114(1):82-96. Epub 2006 Jun 19. Erratum in: Circulation. 2006 Dec 5;114(23):e629. Circulation. 2006 Jul 4;114(1):e27.

63. Nemeroff CB, Evans DL. Correlation between the dexamethasone suppression test in depressed patients and clinical response. *Am J Psychiatry* 1984;141:247–9.

64. Nemeroff CB, Widerlov E, Bissette G, et al. Elevated concentrations of CSF corticotropinreleasing factor-like immunoreactivity in depressed patients. *Science* 1984;226:1342–4.

65. Musselman DL, Tomer A, Manatunga AK, et al. Exaggerated platelet reactivity in major depression. *Am J Psychiatry* 1996;153:1313–7.

66. Musselman DL, Marzec UM, Manatunga A, et al. Platelet Reactivity in Depressed Patients Treated With Paroxetine: Preliminary Findings. *Arch Gen Psychiatry.* 2000;57(9):875–882. doi:10.1001/archpsyc.57.9.875

67. Carney RM, Saunders RD, Freedland KE, Stein P, Rich MW, Jaffe AS. Association of depression with reduced heart rate variability in coronary artery disease. *Am J Cardiol.* 1995 Sep 15;76(8):562–4.

68. Gawaz M., Langer H., May A.E. Platelets in inflammation atherogenesis. *J Clin Invest.* 2005, volume 115, 3378–84.

69. Rozanski A, Blumenthal JA, Kaplan J. Impact of psychological factors on the pathogenesis of cardiovascular disease and implications for therapy. *Circulation.* 1999 Apr 27;99(16):2192–217.

70. Khan SG, Melikian N, Shabeeh H, Cabaco AR, Martin K, Khan F, O'Gallagher K, Chowienczyk PJ, Shah AM. The human coronary vasodilatory response to acute mental stress is mediated by neuronal nitric oxide synthase. *Am J Physiol Heart Circ Physiol.* 2017 Sep 1;313(3):H578-H583. doi: 10.1152/ajpheart.00745.2016. Epub 2017 Jun 23.

71. Preisig M, Waeber G, Mooser V, Vollenweider P. [PsyCoLaus: mental disorders and cardiovascular diseases: spurious association?]. *Rev Med Suisse* 2011;7:2127–9.

72. Chaddha A, Robinson EA, Kline-Rogers E, Alexandris-Souphis T, Rubenfire M. Mental health and cardiovascular disease. *Am J Med* 2016;129: 1145–8.

73. Rugulies R. Depression as a predictor for coronary heart disease: a review and meta-analysis1. *Am J Prev Med* 2002;23:51–61.

74. Denollet J, Maas K, Knottnerus A, Keyzer JJ, Pop VJ. Anxiety predicted premature all-cause and cardiovascular death in a 10-year follow-up of middle-aged women. *J Clin Epidemiol* 2009;62: 452–6.

75. Blumenthal JA, Babyak MA, O'Connor C, Keteyian S, Landzberg J, Howlett J, et al. Effects of exercise training on depressive symptoms inpatients with chronic heart failure: the HF-ACTION randomized trial. *JAMA* 2012;308:465–74.

76. Janszky I, Ahnve S, Lundberg I, Hemmingsson T. Early-onset depression, anxiety, and risk of subsequent coronary heart disease: 37-year follow-up of 49,321 young Swedish men. *J Am Coll Cardiol* 2010;56:31–7.

77. Leenen FHH. Brain mechanisms contributing to sympathetic hyperactivity and heart failure. *Circ Res.* 2007; 101: 221–3.

78. Roest AM, Martens EJ, de Jonge P, Denollet J. Anxiety and risk of incident coronary heart disease: a meta-analysis. *J Am Coll Cardiol* 2010;56: 38–46.

79. Phillips AC, Batty GD, Gale CR, et al. Generalized anxiety disorder, major depressive disorder, and their comorbidity as predictors of all-cause and cardiovascular mortality: the Vietnam experience study. *Psychosom Med* 2009;71:395–403.

80. Rutledge T, Linke SE, Krantz DS, et al. Comorbid depression and anxiety symptoms as predictors of cardiovascular events: results from the NHLBI-sponsored Women's Ischemia Syndrome Evaluation (WISE) study. *Psychosom Med* 2009; 71:958–64.

81. Chida Y, Steptoe A. The association of anger and hostility with future coronary heart disease: a meta-analytic review of prospective evidence. *J Am Coll Cardiol* 2009;53:936–46.

82. Lampert R, Joska T, Burg MM, Batsford WP, McPherson CA, Jain D. Emotional and physical precipitants of ventricular arrhythmia. *Circulation* 2002;106:1800–5.

83. Krantz DS, Kop WJ, Santiago HT, Gottdiener JS. Mental stress as a trigger of myocardial ischemia and infarction. *Cardiology clinics* 1996;14(2):271–87.

84. Krantz DS, McCeney MK. Effects of psychological and social factors on organic disease: a critical assessment of research on coronary heart disease. *Annu Rev Psychol* 2002;53:341–69.

References

85. Karasek R, Baker D, Marxer F, Ahlbom A, Theorell T. Job decision latitude, job demands, and cardiovascular disease: a prospective study of Swedish men. *Am J Publ Health* 1981;71:694–705.

86. Greenlund KJ, Kiefe CI, Giles WH, Liu K. Associations of job strain and occupation with subclinical atherosclerosis: the CARDIA study. Ann Epidemiol 2010;20:323–31.

87. Eller NH, Netterstrøm B, Gyntelberg F, et al. Work-related psychosocial factors and the development of ischemic heart disease: a systematic review. *Cardiol Rev* 2009;17:83–97.

88. Leor J, Poole WK, Kloner RA. Sudden cardiac death triggered by an earthquake. *N Engl J Med* 1996;334:413–9.

89. Ader R; Felten DL; Cohen N, eds. *Psychoneuroimmunology*, Volume 2. Academic Press, 2000.

90. Rosengren A, Hawken S, Ôunpuu S, et al. Association of psychosocial risk factors with risk of acute myocardial infarction in 11 119 cases and 13 648 controls from 52 countries (the INTERHEART study): case-control study. *Lancet* 2004;364: 953–62.

91. Orth-Gomer K, Wamala SP, Horsten M, Schenck-Gustafsson K, Schneiderman N, Mittleman MA. Marital stress worsens prognosis in women with coronary heart disease: the Stockholm Female Coronary Risk Study. *JAMA* 2000; 284:3008–14.

92. Herd J.A., Cardiovascular response to stress. *Physiological Review* 1991, volume 71, 305–30

93. Danesh J., et al. Plasma fibrinogen level and risk of major cardiovascular disease and nonvascular mortality: an individual participant metaanalysis, *JAMA* 2005, volume 294, 1799–1809.

94. Kessler R., et al., Posttraumatic stress disorders in a national comorbidity survey, *Archives of General Psychiatry*, 1995, volume 52, 1048–60.

95. Kubzanski L.D., et al., Prospective study of the posttraumatic stress disorder symptom in coronary artery disease and normative aging study. *Archives of General Psychiatry*, 2007, volume 64, 109–16.

96. von Kanel, et al. Altered blood coagulation in patients with posttraumatic stress disorder. *Psychosomatic Medicine*, 2006, volume 68, 598–604.

97. von Kanel, et al. Measures of endothelial dysfunction in plasma with patients with posttraumatic stress disorder. *Psychiatry Res.* 2008, volume 158, 363–73.

98. Mewisse M.L. et al., Cortisol and posttraumatic stress disorder in adults: systemic review of metaanalysis. *British Journal of Psychiatry*, 2007, 191:387–92.

99. Sack et al., Low respiratory sinus arrhythmia and prolonged psychophysiological arousal in posttraumatic disorder: Heart rate dynamics and individual differences in arousal regulation, *Biological Psychiatry* 2004, volume 55, 284–90.

100. Tracy K.D., Physiology and immunology of the cholinergic antiinflammatory pathway. *J. Clin. Invest.* 2007, volume 117, 289–96.

101. Gabbay FH, Krantz DS, Kop WJ, et al. Triggers of myocardial ischemia during daily life in patients with coronary artery disease: physical and mental activities, anger and smoking. *J Am Coll Cardiol* 1996;27:585–92.

102. Gullette EC, Blumenthal JA, Babyak M, et al. Effects of mental stress on myocardial ischemia during daily life. *JAMA* 1997;277:1521–6.

103. Jiang W, Babyak M, Krantz DS, et al. Mental stress–induced myocardial ischemia and cardiac events. JAMA 1996;275:1651–6.

104. Hammond DC. What is neurofeedback: an update. J Neurother. 2011;15:305-336.

105. Gunkelman, J. D., & Johnstone, J. (2005). *Neurofeedback and the Brain. Journal of Adult Development*, 12, 93–100.

106. Ros, T., The´berge, J., Frewen, P. A., Kluetsch, R., Densmore, M., Calhoun, V. D., & Lanius, R. A.. Mind over chatter: Plastic up-regulation of the fMRI salience network directly after EEG neurofeedback. *Neuroimage*, 2013; 65: 324–35.

107. Zoefel B, Huster RJ, Herrmann CS. Neurofeedback training of the upper alpha frequency band in EEG improves cognitive performance. *Neuroimage.* 2011; 54: 1427–31. doi: 10.1016/j.neuroimage.2010. 08.078

108. Ros T., The´berge J., Frewen P. A., Kluetsch R., Densmore M., Calhoun V. D., et al. Mind over chatter: plastic up-regulation of the fMRI salience network directly after EEG neurofeedback. *Neuroimage.* 2013; 65: 324–335. doi: 10.1016/j.neuroimage.2012.09.046

109. Nicholson A, Rabellino D, Densmore M; Frewen P, Paret C, Kluetsch R. et al The Neurobiology of Emotion Regulation in Posttraumatic Stress Disorder: Amygdala Downregulation via Real-Time fMRI Neurofeedback. *Hum Brain Mapp.* 2017 Jan;38(1):541-560. doi: 10.1002/hbm.23402. Epub 2016 Sep 20.

110. Hammond, D. C. (2005). Neurofeedback with anxiety and affective disorders. *Child Adolescent Psychiatric*, 14(1), 105–23.

111. Vanathy, S., Sharma, P. S. V. N., & Kumar, K. B. (1998). The efficacy of alpha and theta neurofeedback training in treatment of generalized anxiety disorder. *Indian Journal of Clinical Psychology*, 25(2), 136–43.

112. Jarusiewicz, B. Efficacy of neurofeedback for children in the Autistic Spectrum: A pilot study. *Journal of Neurotherapy.* 2002: 6(4): 39–49.

113. Kouijzer, M., de Moor, J. M. H., Gerrits, B. J. L., Congedo, M., & van Schie, H. T. Neurofeedback improves executive functioning in children with autism spectrum disorders. *Research in Autism Spectrum Disorders*, 2009; 3(1): 145–62.

114. Monastra, V. J. Electroencephalographic biofeedback (neurotherapy) as a treatment for attention deficit hyperactivity disorder: Rationale and empirical foundations. *Child and Adolescent Psychiatric Clinics of North America.* 2005 14: 55–82.

115. Monastra, V. J., Lynn, S., Linden, M., Lubar, J. F., Gruzelier, J., & La Vaque, T. J. Electroencephalographic biofeedback in the treatment of attention-deficit/hyperactivity disorder. *Journal of Neurotherapy.* 2006; 9(4): 5–34.

References

116. Steiner N. J., Frenette E. C., Rene K. M., Brennan R. T., & Perrin E. C. In-school neurofeedback training for ADHD: sustained improvements from a randomized control trial. *Pediatrics*, 2014; 133, 483–492. doi: 10.1542/peds.2013–59

117. Linden D. E., Habes I., Johnston S. J., Linden S., Tatineni R., Subramanian L et al Real-time self-regulation of emotion networks in patients with depression. *PLoS One*, 2012; 7(6), e38115. doi: 10.1371/ journal.pone.0038115

118. Sokhadze T. M., Cannon R. L., Trudeau D. L. EEG biofeedback as a treatment for substance use disorders: review, rating of efficacy and recommendations for further research. *Appl. Psychophysiol. Biofeedback*. 2008; 33: 1–28 doi: 10.1007/s10484-007-9047-5

119. Stephanie Maxine Ross. Neurofeedback: An Integrative Treatment of Substance Use *Disorders. Holist Nurs Pract* 2013;27(4):246–50.

120. Dehghani-Arani F, Rostami R, Nadali H. Neurofeedback Training for Opiate Addiction: Improvement of Mental Health and Craving. *Appl Psychophysiol Biofeedback*. 2013; 38: 133–41 DOI 10.1007/s10484-013-9218-5.

121. Kluetsch R. C., Ros T., Theberge J., Frewen P. A., Calhoun V. D., Schmahl C., et al. Plastic modulation of PTSD resting-state networks and subjective wellbeing by EEG neurofeedback. *Acta Psychiatrica Scandinavica*. 2014; 130: 123–36. doi: 10.1111/acps.12229

122. Gapen M., van der Kolk B. A., Hamlin E., Hirshberg L., Suvak M., & Spinazzola J. A Pilot Study of Neurofeedback for Chronic PTSD. *Applied psychophysiology and biofeedback*, 2016; 40, 1–11.

123. Kotchoubey, B., Strehl, U., Uhlmann, C., Holzapfel, S., Konig, M., Froscher, W., et al. Modification of slow cortical potentials in patients with refractory epilepsy: A controlled outcome study. *Epilepsies*. 2001; 42(3), 406–16.

124. Hammond, D. C. (2003). QEEG-guided neurofeedback in the treatment of obsessive compulsive disorder. *Journal of Neurotherapy*, 7(2), 25–52.

125. Gruzelier J. H. EEG-neurofeedback for optimising performance. I: a review of cognitive and affective outcome in healthy participants. *Neuroscience & Biobehavioral Reviews* 2014; 44:124–41.

126. Gruzelier, J. H., Foks, M., Steffert, T., Chen, M. L., & Ros, T. Beneficial outcome from EEG-neurofeedback on creative music performance, attention and well-being in school children. *Biological Psychology*. 2014; 95: 86–95.

127. Ros T., Munneke M. A. M., Parkinson L. A., & Gruzelier J. H. Neurofeedback facilitation of implicit motor learning. *Biological Psychology*. 2014; 95: 54–8. doi: 10.1016/j.biopsycho.2013.04.013.

128. Scott, W. C., Kaiser, D., Othmer, S., & Sideroff, S. I. (2005). Effects of an EEG biofeedback protocol on a mixed substance abusing population. *The American Journal of Drug and Alcohol Abuse*, 3, 1455–69.

129. Kaiser, D. A., & Othmer, S. (2000). Effect of neurofeedback on variables of attention in a large multi-center trial. *Journal of Neurotherapy*, 4(1), 5–28.

130. Demos, J. N. (2005). *Getting started with neurofeedback*. New York, London: Norton & company.

131. Gunkelman, J. D., & Johnstone, J. (2005). Neurofeedback and the Brain. *Journal of Adult Development*, 12, 93–100.

132. Gruzelier J, Egner T. Critical validation studies of neurofeedback. *Child Adolesc Psychiatr Clin N Am.* 2005;14:83–104.

133. Cardinali DP. *Autonomic Nervous System: Basic and Clinical Aspects*. Springer International Publishing AG, 2018.

134. Even N, Devaud JM, and Barron A. General Stress Responses in the Honey Bee. *Insects.* 2012; 3: 1271–98. doi: 10.3390/insects3041271